Improving Patient Outcomes

Also of interest from M&K Publishing.

Books can be ordered online at: www.mkupdate.co.uk

Nurse Facilitated Hospital Discharge
ISBN 978-1-905539-12-6
This book has been written for clinical practitioners and aims to provide a pragmatic insight regarding complex issues in hospitals underpinning facilitated discharges from hospital settings. It is compiled and edited by Liz Lees. Contributors included are from Education, Senior Management, Pharmacy, Medicine, Allied Health Professionals and a range of senior nursing roles.

SKILLS FOR CARING SERIES
Self-directed study workbooks that will appeal to everyone with a health and social care interest. They can be used as a stand-alone modules or part of an assessment programme, or as part of a more formal training programme at a college or in the workplace. They have been designed to be very flexible.

Interpersonal Skills Workbook
ISBN: 978-1-905539-37-6

Loss and Grief Workbook
ISBN: 978-1-905539-43-7

Management of Pain in Older People Workbook
ISBN: 978-1-905539-22-2

Visit the M&K website for a full listing of titles in print and forthcoming books.

A sample of forthcoming titles :

COPD: diagnosis and management in hospital and the community
ISBN: 978-1-905539-28-4

ECG Workbook, The
ISBN: 978-1-905539-14-7

Healthcare Management in Practice: an introductory guide
ISBN: 978-1-905539-33-8

Legal Principles and Clinical Practice
ISBN: 978-1-905539-32-1

Managing Emotions in Women's Health
ISBN: 978-1-905539-07-9

Ward-based Critically Ill Patients: a guide for health professionals
ISBN: 978-1-905539-03-1

Improving Patient Outcomes

A resource for ward leaders

Alison Wells

MSc PGDAE BA(Hons) DPNS RM RGN

ISBN: 978-1-905539-06-2

First published 2007

British Library Catalogue in Publication Data
A catalogue record for this book is available from the British Library

Notice:
Clinical practice and medical knowledge constantly evolve. Standard safety precautions must be followed, but, as knowledge is broadened by research, changes in practice, treatment and drug therapy may become necessary or appropriate. Readers must check the most current product information provided by the manufacturer of each drug to be administered and verify the dosages and correct administration, as well as contraindications. It is the responsibility of the practitioner, utilising the experience and knowledge of the patient, to determine dosages and the best treatment for each individual patient. Neither the publisher nor the authors assume any liability for any injury and/or damage to persons or property arising from this publication.

The Publisher

To contact M&K Publishing write to:
M&K Update Ltd · The Old Bakery · St. John's Street
Keswick · Cumbria CA12 5AS

Tel: 01768 773030 · Fax: 01768 781099
publishing@mkupdate.co.uk
www.mkupdate.co.uk

Designed & typeset in 10pt Usherwood Book by Mary Blood
Printed in England by Ferguson Print (Keswick) Ltd.

Contents

About the author

Alison Wells has worked in an acute hospital settings for most of her career. She became a ward leader in 1989 – a role which she found challenging, rewarding and enjoyable for more than four years.

She moved into practice development where she developed her teaching and facilitation skills. Alison also has experience as a Change Leader delivering workshops on managing transitions, team building and redesign techniques all over the UK. Her most recent role in the NHS has been as Professional Head of Nursing (Education and Research) in an acute trust. There she led a number of projects including developing competencies for nurse practitioners and running a ward leader development programme.

Alison set up Smart Work Consulting in 2005 and has established a successful business working with organisations across the country. Her work includes training and development, strategy development, programme evaluation and event organisation.

Alison is committed to the improvement of patient care and developing people. Everything she does is based on these two principles. Her expertise includes working with teams, strategy development, change management, nurse-led discharge, writing for publication, patient and public involvement, customer care, political awareness, coaching, mentoring and much more.

Introduction

The ward leader has long been recognised as a pivotal role in the effective running of the ward team and the maintenance of high standards of care (King's Fund, 1988; Kitson, 1991; Pembrey 1980). Yet ward leaders are often ill prepared for the role, lack support and time. They report conflicting objectives and priorities (Allen, 2001; Binnie & Titchen, 1998).

This book is aimed at ward leaders and prospective ward leaders. The evidence for effective team working and its impact on patient care is readily available. As a ward leader you do not have to make enormous changes to the way you work to have an effect.

Kotter describes leadership as aligning people, setting the direction, motivating and inspiring people, developing credibility, being visionary, anticipating and coping with change (Kotter, 1990). I hope this book will help you to build on and develop skills in all these areas.

All the chapters link with each other but they also stand alone. You are not expected to work on your own to implement changes but to seek out help from your peers and colleagues within your team and organisation.

Good luck!

Acknowledgements

I would like to thank my husband Tim for his patience and support, here and in France, whilst I wrote this book. I need to thank him for much more, but he knows that.

I would also like to thank my close friends and colleagues who have readily shared their knowledge with me.

Thank you also to Mike who put up with me missing endless deadlines.

Chapter 1
Improving patient outcomes

The nurse's role in relation to patient outcomes

There are numerous misunderstandings and stereotypes of what nurses do. If you put 'nurse' into an internet image search engine you will find nurses in scanty uniforms, or domineering Hatty Jacques-type images and the occasional nurse in theatre garb. None of these capture what nursing is really about. Lots of people have attempted to define nursing, starting with Florence Nightingale, who described nursing as:

> *Nature alone cures ... and what nursing has to do is to put the patient in the best condition for nature to act upon him.*
>
> (Nightingale, 1859)

Virginia Henderson's (1966) definition is one of the best known and most well used:

> *The unique function of the nurse is to assist the individual, sick or well, in the performance of those activities contributing to health or its recovery (or to a peaceful death) that he would perform unaided if he had the necessary strength, will or knowledge ... and to do this in such a way as to help him gain independence as rapidly as possible.*

The International Council of Nurses (ICN) claims that:

> *Nursing encompasses autonomous and collaborative care of individuals of all ages, families, groups and communities, sick or well and in all settings. Nursing includes the promotion of health, prevention of illness, and the care of ill, disabled and dying people. Advocacy, promotion of a safe environment, research, participation in shaping health policy and in patient and health systems management, and education are also key nursing roles.*
> (www.icn.ch/definition.htm)

Improving patient outcomes

Finally the Royal College of Nursing (RCN) published a definition following consultation and discussion with representatives of its members in 2003:

> *Nursing is the use of clinical judgement in the provision of care to enable people to improve, maintain, or recover health, to cope with health problems, and to achieve the best possible quality of life, whatever the disease or disability, until death.*

This definition is supported by six characteristics: mode of intervention, domain, focus, value base, commitment to partnership and purpose.

Between them these definitions paint a picture of nursing as being about assisting, being attentive, reliable, enabling and acting as advocate, as well as about influencing policy. All of them describe the nursing role as one which improves patient outcomes – even Florence Nightingale as long ago as the nineteenth century.

The Healthcare Commission (2005) states:

> *Ward staff spend more time with patients than any other staff group in hospitals. They have a major impact on the experience of patients and the outcomes of their stay in hospital, as well as on the overall efficiency of trusts.*

Nurse managers have a responsibility to ensure the delivery of safe care. This has to be achieved not only during the day-to-day running of a ward but also by using research findings to influence the delivery and organisation of care and by influencing policy making.

Acute trusts spend on average 30% of their budget on staffing wards and yet between 10% and 20% of patients are not happy with their care (based on complaint figures (Healthcare Commission, 2005)).

The National Patient Survey which is carried out across acute trusts by the Picker Institute, on behalf of the Healthcare Commission, demonstrates that most patients are satisfied with their care but there are still areas of concern. In the 2006 survey approximately 40% of the 82,000 respondents felt that there were not enough nurses on duty and there are still patients who do not get the help they need with feeding and those who experience slow responses to call bells.

Improving patient outcomes

There are a number of drivers to improve patient care not least the need to respond to patient expectations. The financial incentive to improve patient outcomes is great. Poor patient outcomes lead to increased length of stay and therefore increased costs. Chief executives have an obligation to 'balance the books' and this is becoming increasingly difficult. In the financial year 2005–6, NHS overspending hit £536 million. This year hospitals and primary care trusts have been told to cut £1 billion (Reuters, 2006). As a result, job cuts have been announced in a number of trusts (Lister, 2006). Nurses, therefore, have a responsibility to ensure that care is delivered economically as well as safely, something which does not always sit well with nurses who strive to give a high standard of care (Bradshaw, 2003; Torjuul, 2006; Forsyth, 2006).

There are many factors that influence the ability of nurses to deliver high quality care. There is also a wealth of evidence to help nurses to improve patient outcomes by ensuring the right factors are in place. Nurses need therefore to be familiar with the research and also how to interpret and implement it, and a number of research texts are available to help nurses develop these skills (Clifford, 2004; Crookes, 2004; Polit, 2004).

Nurses will often complain that there are not enough nurses working a shift. While the nurse to patient ratio is important, research shows that it is not the necessarily the number of nurses working but the skill and experience of those nurses and the ratio of registered nurses to healthcare assistants that matter (RCN, 2002). Other factors include team working and organisational culture.

Nursing numbers

Nursing numbers

Insufficient nurse staffing levels can lead to poor or unsafe care (NHS Executive, 1999). Research undertaken by Aiken (2002) and Rafferty (2006) shows that high patient to nurse ratios can lead to increased risk of patient mortality. For example, post-operative patients are at higher risk of dying (7% for each additional patient per nurse). Clarke (2002) demonstrated that low staffing levels can lead to an increased likelihood of staff sustaining needlestick injuries. Higher nurse staffing levels have also been shown to result in reduced numbers of urinary tract infection, pneumonia and upper gastrointestinal bleeding (ICN, available at www.icn.ch under Factsheets).

Rafferty has also demonstrated that staff in hospitals that have a high patient to staff ratio are likely to be twice as dissatisfied as staff in hospitals with a lower staff to patient ratio. They also report a lower standard of care.

In some parts of the world where this is recognised, nurse to patient ratios are set and are mandatory (parts of America and Australia and all of Belgium). Whilst minimum staffing levels would appear to be a good idea, they can become acceptable levels rather than minimal levels.

It is good practice to review your skill mix and staffing levels regularly, to ensure your team matches the needs of the service. Triggers to undertake a review will include increased staff turnover, increased incident reporting and changes in practice or competence of the team.

There are no national standards for ward staffing in the UK and no formulas to help calculate skill mix and staffing levels. Ward budgets tend to be set using local judgement and cost constraints. There are five broad methods of calculating nurse staffing levels. The most commonly used method is professional judgement, using approaches such as Telford. The Telford approach has three basic stages:

The Telford approach

1. Ward staff set safe and acceptable levels of staff for each shift for each day of the week. They then support this with written evidence and support for their decisions.
2. The numerical assessments are then transposed into bands of staff and whole time equivalents.
3. Actual numbers and bands of staff are summarised and appropriate allowances for trained and permanent staff are built in by managers.

This simple method needs to be supported by audits to ensure that quality of care is delivered.

Other approaches

The *nurses per occupied bed* criterion calculates the average number of staff by grade per bed. The *acuity-quality* method takes into account patient dependency and quality of care, which makes it more complex to calculate but more flexible as you can adjust staffing levels if dependency on the ward changes. The *time task/activity* method looks at the time it takes nurses to complete each task related to patient care. It is a useful method where nursing activity is predictable. Finally, the least used method is the *regression analysis* method which predicts the required number of nurses for a given level of activity (Hurst, 1993). Again, this is useful if you are able to predict activity such as admissions and discharges.

Determining the minimum staffing levels for a ward is complex as you need to take into account not only dependency and numbers of patients but the layout of the ward, the number of discharges and admissions and the skills and abilities of the team members.

There is no one tool which will meet the total needs of any clinical environment. The important thing to remember is that you should not use the tool to dictate your staffing levels but to support the decisions you make. Using a combination of tools may make the information you produce more credible.

Using a tool will establish a baseline that you can use for negotiations with your managers, but it must be based on reliable, comprehensive and up-to-date information.

Skill mix

Skill mix

It is not just numbers of nurses that are important to deliver a high standard of care. Skill mix is also important.

Skill mix has been defined as:

> *The balance between trained and untrained, qualified and unqualified and supervisory and operative staff within a service area as well as between staff groups . . . optimum skill mix is achieved when the desired standard of service is provided, at the minimum cost, which is consistent with the efficient deployment of trained, qualified and supervisory personnel and the maximisation of contributions from all staff members. It will ensure the best possible use of scarce professional skills to maximise the service to clients.*

(Nessling, 1990)

There is evidence that better quality of care will be delivered by higher grades of staff and that where these staff work alongside those with lower grades the variation in quality of care is reduced (RCN, 2002). The RCN reports that the staffing establishments for general NHS wards is on average 62% to 68% registered nurses (RCN, 2006). This has remained unchanged for five years in spite of the increased activity and dependency on wards and the greater bed occupancy. The report recommends a staffing ration of 65% registered nurses to 35% healthcare assistants.

In 2004, the RCN commissioned *The Future Nurse: Evidence of the Impact of Registered Nurses* (West & Rafferty, 2004) which underlines the finding of a direct relationship between the numbers of registered nurses and patient outcomes. Carr-Hill and Jenkins Clarke (cited in Currie *et al.*, 2005) found that the division of tasks between registered and unregistered nurses was unclear and so staff skills were not always used effectively.

Employing more experienced and skilled staff can result in better patient outcomes. A higher number of registered nurses could result in fewer accidents and incidents. Therefore, building your team with more experienced nurses and increasing your skill mix could be better value for money than simply employing more staff (Healthcare Commission, 2005).

Team working

Team working

The importance of team working in healthcare was outlined in the NHS Plan where team working was cited as being vital to patient-centred care (DH, 2000a). Effective team working can be difficult to achieve, particularly in an environment with different professions, people working shifts and a lack of systems to support team working. Multi-disciplinary teams may consist of several different disciplines with different lines of management. However, the evidence is that effective team working leads to better patient and staff outcomes and it is therefore worth trying to achieve.

The Department of Health (DH) commissioned the Healthcare Team Effectiveness Project to determine how multi-disciplinary team working contributes to the quality, efficiency and innovation in the NHS (Borrill *et al.*, 2001). The research was undertaken by five universities over three years. Information was collected from 400 healthcare teams, 7,000 NHS staff and also NHS clients. The research showed that the quality of team working is related to innovation, mental health, death rates and retention of staff.

The factors that improve the quality of team working are:

- team rewards (see Chapter 5)
- clear objectives/targets (see Chapter 9)
- feedback (see Chapter 4)
- training (see Chapter 4)
- physical environment
- organisational climate (see Figure 1.1)
- team size (see Chapter 1)
- leadership (see Chapter 2)
- team member selection (see Chapter 3)
- team building (see Chapter 4)

Figure 1.1

Organisational climate

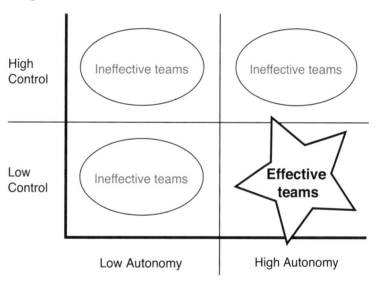

There were a number of findings as a result of the research, relating to both staff and patients.

Staff

Staff

Working in effective teams leads to reduced stress levels among staff. Being a member of a team acts as a buffer against the organisational culture. So, if the organisation you work in has a blame or bullying culture, you can protect your team members from that atmosphere by creating a more positive environment for your team. Poor training, inadequate levels of resources and co-operation and a lack of individual feedback will lead to increased stress levels.

Clear individual and team objectives lead to increased staff retention. Working in an effective team leads to better mental health for staff. Borrill and West (2001) have shown that team nursing can lead to a reduction in sick leave.

Patients

Patients

A related study carried out at the Aston Centre for Health Service Organisation Research (cited in Borrill *et al.*, 2001) shows that the more people who work in teams in trusts, the lower the number of patient deaths (as measured by the Sunday Times 'Dr Foster' mortality index). This supports the report by the National Confidential Enquiry into Perioperative Deaths (2002) which said that patients could be dying unnecessarily because of a lack of team working. Borrill and West also showed that team nursing can lead to reduced costs per patient stay and reduced length of stay.

Organisational culture

Organisational culture

Magnet hospitals were an initiative were developed in the US in the 1980s. Those hospitals awarded Magnet status were identified as successful at recruiting, retaining and motivating nursing staff. Research carried out into those hospitals has demonstrated benefits to patient outcomes which include increased patient satisfaction with care, fewer complications and lower mortality rates. Benefits to nursing staff are higher levels of job satisfaction, lower levels of burnout and fewer nurse reported needlestick injuries (NHRSU, 2006).

The characteristics of Magnet hospitals are that they have a participatory and supportive management style, the nurse executives are well prepared for the role and there is a decentralised structure, adequate staffing and flexible rostering. Staff have clear career opportunities and are professionally autonomous and responsible.

The criteria required for organisations to qualify for Magnet status are:

- Nurses monitor and evaluate the needs of clients (see Chapter 8).
- There is patient-centred care planning.
- There is continuous improvement of clinical guidelines and these are linked to patient outcomes.
- Staff participate in teams.
- Educational activities for staff are promoted.
- Performance appraisals are undertaken.
- Research is undertaken.
- Effective communication is in place.
- Nurses use nursing quality indicators.

To promote Magnet hospital characteristics in your team, you need to encourage professional accountability by allowing nurses to act on their expert judgement. Encourage nurses to participate in writing and reviewing evidence-based policies. Implement a decision-making structure (see www.mindtools.com and follow the link to Decision Making). Promote and recognise excellent nursing practice. Provide educational and career support (see Chapter 4) and encourage team working with the medical staff (NHSRU, 2006).

Chapter 2

Diagnosis: how well is your team performing?

This chapter is designed to help you identify who your team are and how well they work together as a team. It introduces several tools and techniques to help you with this; some are easier to use than others. You may wish to talk to your practice development team or your human resources department to see whether they have anyone who can help you to use them until you feel confident to go it alone.

What is a team?

What is a team?

There are numerous definitions of a team; Mohrman *et al.* define a team as:

> *A group of individuals who work together to produce products or deliver services for which they are mutually accountable. Team members share goals and are mutually held accountable for meeting them, they are interdependent in their accomplishment, and they affect the results through their interactions with one another. Because the team is held collectively accountable, the work of integrating with one another is included among the responsibilities of each member.*
>
> (Mohrman *et al.*, 1995)

Who belongs to your team?

In healthcare the membership of teams varies enormously. You may regard your team as consisting of nursing staff only or you may include the medical staff or the entire multi-disciplinary team (social workers, physiotherapists and so on). There are no rules as to whom you should include and whom you shouldn't.

Improving patient outcomes

Cross-functional team working (team working across professional and/or organisational boundaries) tends to work best when working on a specific problem over a limited period of time, rather than ongoing work.

You might want to consider cross-functional working when you are developing protocols or practices that involve other professionals or people from other organisations or departments. Some examples are:

- implementing nurse-led discharge
- developing care pathways
- implementing multi-disciplinary meetings
- developing patient information.

When considering who your long-term team are you need to think about the following factors:

Span of control – If you are going to work with your 'team' to improve their performance you need to have some influence over the members of that team. Your span of control will depend on the number of people who report directly and indirectly to you. The smaller the span of your control, the more you will be able to supervise those you manage but the less you will be able to influence those you don't. If you are directly responsible for a large team you will not have such a close relationship with your team members and you will have less influence.

Level of interaction – The amount of interaction you have with individuals of the team and the feedback that takes place between yourself and others.

The location of the workers – For example if you work in primary care and your team work in different locations your ability to influence them will be less.

Your style of leadership – This is discussed later in this chapter. Your style of leadership may help you overcome other obstacles, particularly if you have strong negotiation, motivation and influencing skills.

Support from people you do not directly manage – If there are people in the 'extended' team who will help you achieve your goals then use them. You will need all the help you can get.

The Nursing and Midwifery Council (NMC) code of conduct (2002) states that:

> as a registered nurse, midwife, or health visitor, you must co-operate with others in the team

and that:

> the team includes the patient or client, the patient's or client's family, informal carers and health and social care professionals in the National Health Service, independent and voluntary sectors.

Whilst there is a need to work with this group of people, for the sake of developing an effective clinical team, you may wish to focus on the ward team in the first instance.

Figure 2.1 **Defining team membership**

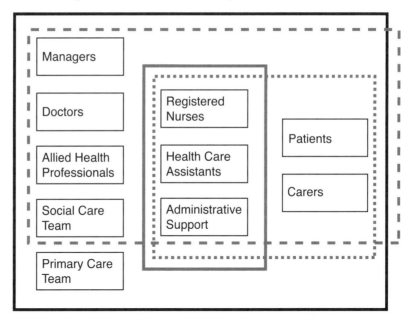

Figure 2.1 shows how you might determine membership of your team. Don't forget to include support staff such as administrative staff, housekeepers and hostesses. They are the people who can provide influence and an in-depth knowledge of the organisation (Modernisation Agency, 2004). Remember to consider the impact of what you are doing on the wider team, particularly those people that you don't include. It is good practice to incorporate patient and public involvement in any service changes you make, so you may want to seek their views early on when developing your team (see Chapter 8).

Once you have determined who you are including in your team you can begin to look at how they work together.

Stages of team development

Team Development

Bruce Tuckman first described four stages of team development in 1965 and, although now more than 40 years old, his analysis is still relevant to team development today (Tuckman, 1965).

When teams come together they go through the following stages:

- forming
- storming
- norming
- performing.

Forming

At the forming stage teams question their purpose, the role of the manager or team leader and roles and responsibilities are unclear. This stage occurs when a team first comes together to work in a particular way, this may be because a new member has joined or because of a situational change. Team members begin to form opinions about each other – whom they like or dislike. The outcomes of this stage are that the members get to know each other and start to develop commitment to the team.

Storming

Storming takes place as the team starts to organise itself. Clashes may occur as the purpose of the team becomes clearer but member's interpretations differ. Politeness can be dropped a little as the team are getting to know each other. Friction may occur which makes team working difficult and it can ultimately lead to the team's failure if the situation isn't managed. It is at this stage that teams need to be clear about their goals. You will need to spend time finding out what individuals' concerns and feelings are and provide one-to-one sessions with team members.

Although it is unusual, teams can get stuck in the storming stage. If you think this might be happening get help as soon as you can. You can get support from your practice development department, human resources or using an external facilitator.

Norming

In the norming stage, the team becomes much clearer about roles and responsibilities and starts to make big decisions. Communication systems are developing, both informal and formal. Team members also become more motivated and committed. Teams may regress from time to time to the storming stage but this should occur less frequently over time. You will still need to give direction during this stage to prevent this regression and to avoid complacency if the team is doing well.

Performing

The team becomes more effective; they are autonomous and can resolve conflicts themselves. Problems are solved jointly; confidence and levels of trust are high. This is the stage at which the team is most highly motivated.

This model is cyclical. Teams may not stay at the performing stage indefinitely; in fact the nature of nursing work means that you may quite often return to the forming stage. The important thing is to recognise which stage you are at and what interventions you should make.

Recognising the stages

Recognising the stages

Forming

This stage is likened to being at a cocktail party. It is the polite stage where everyone is trying to get to know everyone else. The team is generally positive although this may be because they are being polite and do not wish to offend.

There may be some anxiety as people are getting to know each other and understand their role. They will be concerned about whether they fit in.

Storming

You will witness power struggles and conflict. Members will complain about the way the team has been established and how members have been recruited. This will be a tense period. You and the members will be frustrated. It is unlikely you will be achieving your targets or goals.

Norming

The team will start to blame each other less. There is more discussion and debate and more decision making. People will start to think of the team rather than themselves; they may even be telling others what a great team they work for.

Performing

If you have performance measures in place, you will be achieving them! Members will be confident and will be challenging each other but in the right way. They will be supporting each other and any disagreements will be handled in a positive and mature way.

It can be very difficult for a team leader to assess which stage their team is at, but it is highly important as you will not be able to provide the right level of support unless you know where they are. Donald Clark has created a Team Work Survey which will help you make a more accurate assessment (Appendix 2).

Leadership styles

Leadership styles

The role of the team leader is to influence the team toward a common goal. This may be your philosophy or vision and will incorporate your performance measures (see Chapter 9).

You will need to use different leadership styles to cope with each of the stages. Hersey and Blanchard (1977) offer a model that you can adopt. Their model of situational leadership describes four different styles (see Figure 2.2).

'Telling' is the style you should adopt if team members' commitment and motivation is low and also if they are not familiar with their roles. It is therefore a style you can adopt when your team is at the forming stage. You will need to give clear direction, make decisions, and set boundaries.

'Selling' or coaching is a more supportive approach which you can use when the team needs to have more focus; this is a helpful style to use when the team is storming. You will need to continue to clarify roles and the purpose of the team, however you can begin to include members in some of the decision making while retaining the final say. If you can keep the team focused on patient needs this will help. Ensure you act as a role model as team members will still be assessing the boundaries for their behaviour. When the team is norming you can take on a 'participating' style and use facilitative skills to encourage the team to take on more responsibility. Encourage group members to resolve conflicts themselves and take a step back. Having the confidence to do this can be difficult. It's very much like letting your children start taking responsibility for themselves. You have to let go to enable them to learn. It is the only way your team will move to the performing stage.

Figure 2.2   **Situational leadership**

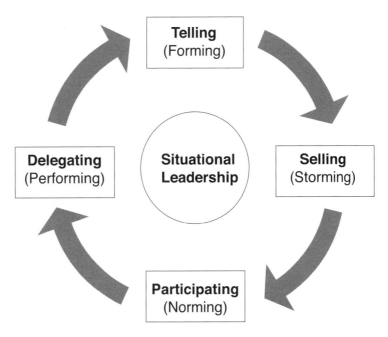

(Based on Hersey and Blanchard, 1977)

Once the team reaches the performing stage you can delegate responsibility to them as they have gained competence and confidence in their roles. You can now set long-term goals; you also need to start giving rewards for performance (see Chapter 5).
The style of leadership you adopt will need to change to fit the situation. Therefore you need to be aware of what is happening in your team and be flexible with your approach.

Other diagnostic tools

Other diagnostic tools

There are a number of other tools you can use to diagnose how well your team is working together.

In 2005, the Royal College of Nursing (RCN) published *Working with Care: Improving Working Relationships in Healthcare* (RCN, 2005). This document contains a set of tools which are designed to minimise negative behaviours and maximise positive behaviours in teams at any level of the organisation. You should be experienced in handling sensitive group situations and be independent of the team in order to use the tools, so you may wish to co-opt the help of someone from your training and development department, human resources or an external facilitator to work with you and your team. The document, along with the tools, can be downloaded from the RCN website at www.rcn.org.uk.

Other tools you can use include Belbin and Myers Briggs. The Myers Briggs tool (www.myersbriggs.org) measures your inborn preferences. Isabel Briggs Myers and her mother Katherine Cook Briggs first published the model in 1975. It is based on Carl Jung's psychological theory. It is designed to help you understand the similarities and differences in the personalities of your team members. It focuses on four preferences: where you prefer to direct your energy (extraversion and introversion); how you prefer to process information (sensing or intuition); how you prefer to organise your life (judging and perception); and how you prefer to make decisions (thinking and feeling). These four preferences give a combination of 16 different types. Once you have identified the preferences of your team and the areas where you can maximise potential you will be able to help your team function better.

Belbin's model (www.belbin.com) helps you to identify team roles which Dr Meredith Belbin defines as:

> *a tendency to behave, contribute and interrelate with others in a particular way.*

Dr Belbin studied the behaviour of managers from all over the world for nine years and identified clusters of roles:

> *Shaper, Implementer, Completer Finisher, Co-Coordinator, Team Worker, Resource Investigator, Plant, Monitor Evaluator, and Specialist.*

Once you have identified the spread of clusters within your team you can start to understand the team dynamics.

Most organisations will employ people who are able to carry out a Myers Briggs or Belbin assessment as well as a number of others for your team, or you can access the respective websites.

Fundamental factors for effective team working

Effective team working

To enable team development you will require some fundamental factors to be in place:

- effective leadership
- shared objectives
- well-defined roles
- an organisational identity
- a purpose – the way the team performs impacts on others
- appropriate team composition
- systems to ensure efficient decision making
- an understanding of what patients and users want from you
- systems of measurement
- effective communication systems.

Borrill and West (2001) provide a number of self-assessment tools to help you to diagnose your own strengths and weaknesses and to assess where your team is.

Effective team work will allow you to become more productive and it will help both individuals and the team as a whole achieve their goals and objectives. More importantly, enabling your team to work well together will lead to improved patient care (Borrill *et al.*, 2001).

The remaining chapters of this book will discuss the fundamental factors for effective teams and help you build on the work you have done diagnosing the stage your team is at.

Chapter 3
Selecting team members

In the recent past, many trusts have had problems recruiting and retaining staff, with turnover rates varying (Healthcare Commission, 2005).

Although there has been a 23% growth in the NHS nursing workforce since 1997, this has not been sufficient to end all staff shortages (RCN, 2005a). In order to keep the workforce constant it is estimated that the profession needs to double the number of students it recruits to counterbalance the number of nurses expected to retire in the next ten years (Parish, 2005). However, in 2005 over 150 trusts have reported financial difficulties and 39% of those said that they had frozen recruitment (RCN, 2005a) and the overspend in a number of trusts has led to redundancies. The impact nationally is difficult to ascertain. In the past the temptation for managers has been to recruit whoever they can in order to fill vacancies. However there is a cost to recruiting the wrong person. It is estimated that British companies waste £12 billion a year because of recruitment mistakes, that's a fifth of the entire annual National Health Service budget (Gribben, 2004). But as well as the financial costs there are others which include:

- disgruntled staff
- less satisfied customers/patients
- increased time supporting and/or training the individual
- greater reliance on other staff members to carry out the work
- less motivation
- increased risks of mistakes.

On top of this you may well have to repeat the whole recruitment process when the individual leaves or when other members of the team leave because morale is low.

The purpose of the recruitment and selection process is to enable you to choose the person who will contribute the most to your team, both in the present and in the future.

All organisations will have their own policies covering the recruitment and selection procedure and each will have a human resources team who are the experts in recruitment and selection and employment practices. It is essential that you work within your organisation's policy as this will not only outline their expectations but will ensure that you comply with the law. You should also refer to your human resources team if you are inexperienced at recruiting staff or if you encounter any difficulties. Local policies will include any training requirements there are for staff who are taking part in the recruitment and selection process. There are also a number of pieces of legislation relating to employment which you need to be aware of:

- Employment Relations Act 2004
- Employment Equality (Sex Discrimination) Regulations 2005 (SI 2005/2467)
- Disability Discrimination Act 2005
- European Working Time Directive.

New roles

New roles

When a member of the team leaves you have an opportunity to think about new ways of working. You do not necessarily have to replace like with like.

First of all, look at what currently happens within your team. What is patient feedback like? Are there parts of the service that need improving? Are there gaps in the day when you could do with more people on duty? Could you replace an unqualified member of staff with a qualified nurse? Evidence shows that the higher the ratio of qualified nurses to unqualified staff results the higher the standard of care (see Chapter 1). Are there tasks being carried out by one person when they could more appropriately be carried out by someone else?

Involve your team in the discussions and obtain patient feedback. If you keep patient focused you are more likely to come up with the right ideas. Don't forget to consider patient safety.

Selecting team members

You don't have to be radical – changing the hours for the post might be sufficient – but don't be afraid to be creative either. Consider what training the post-holder will need, how the individual will fit into the team, what the purpose of the role will be, how you will evaluate its effectiveness and whether it will be a long-term position or might develop into something else. Once you have designed the new role you will need to develop a job description and think about recruitment. The recruitment and selection process includes a number of steps (Figure 3.1).

Figure 3.1

The Recruitment and Selection Process

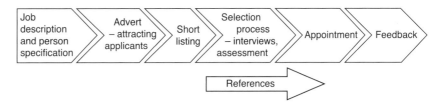

The NHS Employers website also provides useful information about recruiting staff (www.nhsemployers.org).

Job description and person specification

Job description

Before you advertise a post you must ensure you have an up-to-date and accurate job description. The job description describes the role the employee will undertake. It acts as a tool for recruitment and selection as well as a tool for communicating your expectations to the employee.

The job description should be clear, concise and accurate. Your organisation may have a set format which will help ensure that you include everything. Headings will include: title, pay, where the job is based, line management and accountability and the purpose of the job.

The Agenda for Change website (www.dh.gov.uk) includes a number of national job profiles which will help you write job descriptions. It will also help to ensure that you develop a job description that is in keeping with the Agenda for Change framework and so can be easily assessed.

Once you have a job description you need to draw up a person specification. This is a profile of the skills and aptitudes required to do the job. It is important that you have this before you start the selection process as it will contain the criteria by which all applicants can be measured.

The criteria must be divided into those which are essential and those which are desirable. Essential criteria are the minimum that the applicant needs in order to carry out the job. Everyone who is short-listed must meet these criteria. Desirable criteria are needed in the event that more than one candidate meets the essential criteria, these can then be taken into account. Any criteria not included in the person specification should not be taken into account. For example, if the candidate has a degree but this is not included as a requirement for the job, then you cannot favour the candidate because they are a graduate.

The person specification must be an objective tool by which you can assess prospective employees and therefore each criterion must be measurable. For example, you should not include 'must have a good sense of humour' as this can only be assessed subjectively and so is not suitable for inclusion in a person specification. Examples of suitable criteria are included in Table 3.1.

Table 3.1

Criteria for person specification

Knowledge and Skills	Essential	Desirable
Is competent to administer intravenous therapy	*	
Can communicate effectively with others	*	
Ability to communicate clearly in writing	*	
Awareness of current professional nursing issues		*
Ability to adapt to change within working situation		*
Experience		
Experience working in an acute hospital setting		*
Experience working in cardiology		*
Qualifications		
Completed Registered Nurse training	*	
Registered with NMC	*	
Personal attributes		
Can demonstrate continuing professional development	*	

Attracting staff

Attracting staff

If you want to recruit the best staff you need to consider what your area has to offer that others do not. Talk to your existing staff and find out what it is they like about working for you. If you have had problems recruiting you may want to consider some creative approaches, such as offering flexible hours, rotation schemes, new roles (Ambrose, 2002; Baker, 2005). Look in the job sections of journals and see what other areas are offering. Can you match them? Is there anything you can do to make people want to come and work with you? Do you offer training and development, mentorship or clinical supervision? How much support will the individual get when they join you?

Retention of staff starts at this point. Job satisfaction is linked to expectation, so don't offer something which you or your organisation cannot deliver.

You don't always need to advertise externally. Think about current members of your team and whether any of them will meet the person specification. It is important that you allow your own team members the opportunity to develop their career. There may also be individuals working elsewhere in the organisation who will meet your needs. You can advertise internally by using flyers, the intranet and notices.

If you want to advertise the post externally, consult your human resources team or recruitment department as they will be able to help you with the design and wording. A good advertisement should be clear and indicate:

- the role and what the post-holder is required to do
- the necessary and the desirable criteria for job applicants (person specification)
- a description of the area/organisation (for example, dermatology ward in an acute hospital)
- where the post is based
- pay and bonuses
- length of contract (if temporary)
- details of how to apply.

There is a simple acronym to help you write your advert: 'AIDA' or Attention, Interest, Desire and Action.

Attention

Think about the headline for your advert. Again, looking through professional journals may help you, but you need something that will attract the attention of the reader.

Interest

The advert should go on to give the reader information in an interesting way. Readers will only scan the advert for a few seconds, so you need to grab their interest in that time.

Desire

You need to point out the benefits to the reader of coming to work with you. This will not just be down to pay. Other benefits might be:

- Is it a career development opportunity for the reader?
- How much responsibility will they have?
- Is the hospital developing new services?
- Will they be given additional training?
- What staff benefits does the organisation offer – such as a pension scheme, sports and leisure facilities, flexible working, on-site nurseries, holiday play schemes, childcare vouchers or free counselling?

Action

Finally, you need to invite the reader to telephone, email or write. If they can take action quickly whilst you have their interest and desire then all the better. If you invite them to phone make sure there is an answer phone or that you return the call quickly. If you give an email address make sure you're not 'out of office'. If possible give them the opportunity to download an application pack from the hospital website.

An advert in a national journal is expensive but it can have a much wider readership so it is important to get it right. Don't rush this stage. A good response will pay dividends.

Selection

Shortlisting

Once you have successfully attracted people to apply for your post you will need to shortlist them using the person specification. This should be a systematic process and must be carefully documented. Applications should be treated confidentially and only shared with the people taking part in the selection process.

The purpose of shortlisting is to eliminate any unsuitable applicants and to identify those who best meet the criteria for the post. At least two people should participate in the shortlisting process and as many people from the interview panel as possible. Anyone who may prejudice the outcome should be excluded. For example, anyone who is related to any of the applicants should not participate. Each person should individually assess the applications and record their decision. Check whether your organisation has a 'shortlist for interview' form. This will help you maintain a structured approach.

The assessment should be made against the criteria in the person specification and should be based on the application form only. Handwriting, grammar and presentation of the application form should only be taken into account if this is relevant to the post. The purpose of shortlisting is not to compare applicants. Once each individual has made their assessment the panel should come together to make a collective decision. This must be recorded carefully so that feedback can be given to the unsuccessful applicants if they request it.

The lead person must ensure there is no discriminatory practice, referring to human resources or occupational health if the person meets the criteria but there are other reasons that you feel the applicant may not be able to undertake the role due to ill health or disability for example. You may wish to complete the 'self-assessment equalities checklist' at www.equality-online.org.uk to check your practice.

Selection methods

There are a number of methods of selecting the right individual to join your team. These include interviewing, presentations, assessment centres and psychological testing. You may wish to use a combination of these.

Informal visits

Informal visits

These should not be used as part of the selection process but are an important way for the applicant to find out about the organisation, your team and the patient group. Applicants should be encouraged to visit if it is geographically possible. You may also want to give them the opportunity to work a shift or part of a shift. Check your organisation's policy on this. Allowing the applicant to experience as much as possible about the role will help to manage their expectations.

Interviews

Interviews

Interviews are the most commonly used technique for selecting staff, but if they are carried out by untrained people or are unstructured they are a very poor way of testing someone's suitability for a post (CIPD, 2005). Your organisation will have identified the training you need in the recruitment policy, as well as providing guidelines on how to structure the interview.

The aim of an interview is to gather as much information about the candidate as possible so that you can make an objective and accurate assessment of their capabilities.

You will need to consider who will sit on the interview panel. This will usually be the line manager and any other key stakeholders, for example a matron, a representative from human resources or someone in a practice development role.

Plan the interview questions in advance. They should be designed to assess the competencies you are looking for. Your organisation may have a scoring template for you to use. (See Appendix 1 for an example.)

Assessment centres

Assessment centres

Assessment centres were originally used by the War Office following the First World War. An assessment centre is a process comprising a number of activities that replicate the tasks and demands of the post. The idea is to give a rounded evaluation of the candidate's abilities. Research shows that they are more effective than interviews as they help to identify individuals who will fit in with the team (Beagrie, 2004).

The different activities might consist of group discussions, scenarios, simulations, role play and case studies. A range of activities might be needed to assess the range of competencies. An assessment centre can last from a few hours up to two days, depending on the seniority of the post and the investment you want to make.

The observers for the exercise should be briefed and familiar with objective observation techniques. There may be people within your organisation who are trained assessors or you can use external agencies.

Psychometric testing

Psychometric testing

Psychometric testing

There are a number of different psychometric tests. Many are available online for you to try and some are free. Psychometric tests can either be tests of aptitude or personality. Personality tests are the most commonly used. The word 'test' is misnomer. The candidate cannot pass or fail. The tests are an assessment of their attitudes, intelligence and values. Administering and assessing the tests is a skilled process and should only be carried out by someone qualified to do it.

If you decide to use a psychometric test you will need to determine what weighting the test will have as part of the selection process. If the candidate passes the other parts of the selection process but the results of the test do not meet your needs, will you still recruit them?

You will need to consider which test to use and whether it is valid. Benefits of psychometric testing are that it gives you more information about the candidate that may not be revealed by other methods.

Presentations

Presentations

Presentations

It is now common practice to ask candidates to make a presentation as part of the selection process. You need to consider why you want the candidates to make a presentation and what it is that you are trying to assess. You can either give the candidates a presentation title in advance, allowing them time to research the subject and prepare the presentation, or you can give them the title just before you ask them to make the presentation. The latter will help you assess their knowledge as well as their presentation skills whereas the former will assess their presentation skills and their ability to gather evidence on a subject.

Improving patient outcomes

Before appointment

There are several things you must check before appointing the successful candidate.

References

References

Your organisation will have a policy about the uptake of references. It is usual to take these up before appointment, however it is possible to make a provisional offer dependent on good references. Written references must be obtained, but if you need clarification you can telephone the referee. The reference must include details about the applicant's work ability, professional competence and personal qualities – although you need to bear in mind that the latter will be subjective. If there are any gaps in the candidate's employment ask for explanations. It is good practice to tell the candidate when you are going to send for references as they may not have told their current employer that they are looking for work elsewhere.

If you are asked to give a reference for a member of your team, guidelines are included in Appendix 3.

Registration

Registration

If the post is for a registered nurse you must check with the Nursing and Midwifery Council (NMC) that they are on the professional register. Checking their registration card is not sufficient.
The NMC has three methods for you to check registration, online at www.nmc-uk.org, by telephone to a confirmation hotline (24 hours a day, 7 days a week) and by post. You need to verify:

- the applicant's identity (check passport or birth certificate)
- that they have a work permit (for an overseas applicant)
- that the applicant has an up-to-date Criminal Records Bureau check (depending on your organisation's policies and procedures)
- the applicant's qualifications.

Feedback

Giving feedback

Having put candidates through an assessment process, no matter which method you use, you will need to give each of them feedback. Most people prefer giving feedback to the successful candidate. Giving the news to unsuccessful candidates is less enjoyable but nonetheless extremely important.

There are some important points to remember when giving feedback to unsuccessful candidates:

- The feedback should be objective and based on the criteria that you used in the assessment.
- It should be based on the notes made by the panel members.
- Remember to tell them about the things they did well.
- When you tell them about where they didn't meet the criteria, help them identify ways to overcome this in the future.
- If possible give the feedback face to face.

Finally, don't forget to ask them for feedback about the selection process. This will help you and the panel to improve your skills.

Appointment

Appointment

Once you have chosen the successful candidate you will need to set up an induction programme and identify a mentor or clinical supervisor to support them. You will find more information on this in Chapter 4.

Keeping staff once you have appointed them

Keeping staff

Staff turnover in health is 14.1% which equates to 1 in 7 employees leaving. The vast majority (9.2%) will be voluntary leavers (CIPD, 2005b). Staff turnover has high costs in terms of recruitment, loss of skills, utilising temporary staff whilst the vacancy is filled, low morale and induction. A low staff turnover can also be detrimental in that it can cause a lack of promotional opportunities and the retention of poor performers as well as a lack of creativity within the team. The financial cost of staff turnover is estimated to be £4,625 per leaver in 2004 (CIPD, 2005a). For this reason, national policies, The NHS Plan and Improving Working Lives all include initiatives to retain nurses such as flexible working and facilities for childcare as well as the outline for Agenda for Change.

It is important to measure your staff turnover to benchmark your team over a period of time or against other teams. You can calculate it by counting the number of people who have left the team over a certain period of time dividing this by the number of staff that were working in that period and multiplying by 100:

$$\frac{\text{number of leavers}}{\text{number of staff working}} \times 100 = \text{staff turnover rate}$$

This is the formula used nationally and will enable you to make comparisons, but you may want to refine it for your own purposes to include only voluntary leavers, rather than all staff leaving.

Studies undertaken into why nurses leave their roles generally show the reasons to be:

- a poor working environment
- poor quality of patient care due to low staffing levels
- low pay
- stress
- understaffing
- high acuity patients
- number of hours worked.

(Joshua-Amadi, 2003; Strachota, 2003)

Studies which show why nurses stay in their job give the following reasons:

- job satisfaction
- a positive environment
- recognition
- flexibility.

Job satisfaction comes from factors such as extended roles, patient contact and diversity. A key element of a positive working environment includes feeling part of a cohesive team in a supportive environment with a strong leader. (This is covered in more detail in Chapters 2 and 4.) Nurses participate in decision making and there are good working relationships with a manager who has a facilitative style (O'Brien-Pallas *et al.*, 2006)

When nurses talk about recognition for what they do, they do not always mean pay. Many will say that they appreciate being thanked. What they also appreciate is the opportunity for learning and career development (see Chapter 4). Finally, nurses appreciate the opportunity to be able to work flexibly. While they know that they have to work shifts and unsocial hours, if they can adapt their working hours to maintain a better work-life balance this will increase their job satisfaction.

All of these factors are interconnected. Magnet hospitals in the US have shown that where hospitals can demonstrate high staff satisfaction, staff retention is greater and patient mortality is less than the national average (Buchan *et al.*, 2003).

Magnet hospitals suggest the following strategies to increase job satisfaction:

● Promote accountability by allowing nurses to use their expert judgement in clinical situations.
● Encourage nurses to participate in developing and reviewing policies and procedures.
● Recognise excellence and clinical competence.
● Provide educational and career development.
● Enhance your skill mix.
● Encourage multi-disciplinary working.

(NHSRU, 2006)

It isn't realistic to expect to be able to resolve all issues in the short term but there are some basic things you can do to encourage staff to stay:

● say 'thank you'
● create a strong team (see Chapter 2)
● plan off duty in advance, make it flexible and encourage staff to swap shifts if necessary
● encourage learning (see Chapter 4)
● avoid a long hours culture
● do not discriminate or favour certain employees.

Chapter 4
Creating and sustaining a learning environment

Employees value learning opportunities and will choose jobs that offer training and development and organisations that have a learning culture. Studies into why nurses stay in their posts show that education is important to them throughout their careers (see Chapter 4).

In a learning environment:

- people in the team take responsibility for, and support, each other
- team members share experiences
- people learn from their mistakes and successes
- ideas are listened to
- there is a climate of trust.

(Maccoby, 2003)

Attracting and keeping staff are not the only reasons for creating and maintaining a learning environment. Other important drivers include:

- professional regulations
- patient safety
- clinical governance
- Agenda for Change.

Professional regulations

Professional regulations

The Nursing and Midwifery Council (NMC) requires all registered nurses to practice competently. As a registered nurse you must possess the knowledge, skills and abilities required for lawful, safe, effective practice, without direct supervision. You must acknowledge the limits of your professional competence and only undertake practice and accept responsibilities for those activities where you are competent (NMC, 2002: S9).

You are also required to protect patients or clients from coming to harm as a result of someone else's incompetence (NMC, 2002: S11). Lack of competence is defined as:

> a lack of knowledge, skill or judgement of such a nature that a registrant is unfit to practise safely and effectively, in the field in which they claim to be qualified to practise or seek to practise.
>
> Competence should be measured and reassessed regularly and practice should be adjusted accordingly. This means that skills and knowledge should be tested on a regular basis. This should all be recorded in the individual's records

Patient safety

Patient safety

The NHS treats approximately one million patients a day and it is estimated that 10% of those are harmed unintentionally (Beckford-Ball, 2005). The Bristol Inquiry brought patient safety firmly onto the agenda in the mid-1990s. The report of that inquiry gives an account of the events and their background (DH, 2001). The Bristol Royal Infirmary had a service offering paediatric heart surgery across two sites. There were no dedicated intensive care beds for children and no full-time cardiac surgeons. There were also insufficient paediatric nurses. The culture of the service was one of an imbalance of power. Nationally there were no standards of care and vulnerable children were not given a priority. As a result, one-third of children in the service were not given adequate care and between 30 and 35 more children under the age of one year died than might have been expected in a typical unit in England.

Amongst the 200 recommendations from the report there are many principles which can be transferred to other areas of practice including:

- putting patients at the centre of care and service delivery
- rooting out unsafe practices
- ensuring staff have the right competencies
- establishing clear lines of accountability for all staff
- maintaining high standards of care
- promoting a culture of openness and honesty.

Creating and sustaining a learning environment

Both the National Audit Office (NAO, 2005) and the National Patient Safety Agency (NPSA) have identified a lack of openness and a blame culture as a factor. A breakdown in communication is cited as a reason for many incidents. In order to overcome this it is recommended that staff have regular appraisals and that organisations develop a learning culture.

As a manager and registered nurse you therefore have an obligation to ensure that each member of your team is developed and assessed on a regular basis. In order to achieve this, they will need to be appraised.

Clinical governance

Clinical governance

Clinical governance is defined as:

> *a framework through which NHS organisations are accountable for continually improving the quality of their services and safeguarding high standards of care by creating an environment in which excellence in clinical care will flourish.*

(Scally & Donaldson, 1998)

The events at Bristol Infirmary, resulting in the Bristol Inquiry (DH, 2001) had an influence on the implementation of clinical governance.

There are several components to clinical governance, including:

- clinical effectiveness
- risk management
- patient experience
- communication
- resource management
- strategic effectiveness
- learning
- systems awareness
- team work
- leadership
- patient and public involvement.

Essentially clinical governance has been put in place to help organisations learn from one another and therefore improve the quality of patient care. It is about promoting a learning culture and promoting innovation. All NHS Trusts have a statutory obligation to implement and maintain the clinical governance framework. All will have someone working at board level with the responsibility for clinical governance. There will also be people in the organisation with roles related to the components outlined above. If you don't already know who these people are, find out. They will be able to help you implement the changes in practice that you want to make.

Nurses have a key role in clinical governance as the central theme is the patients' experience and they are in a position to influence many aspects of their care.

Phipps (2000) identifies six questions you should ask yourself and your team members to help them reflect on clinical governance and their practice.

- Do I reflect on my practice
  (perhaps with a clinical supervisor or mentor)?
- Am I using the most up-to-date evidence to influence the care I give?
- Am I involved in auditing the care the patients receive?
- Am I involving my patients in their care planning and delivery?
- Am I confident about raising concerns about patient care?
- Is my personal development plan based on service need as well as personal aspirations?

You can use these questions to help your team members identify their learning needs.

Agenda for Change

Agenda for Change

Agenda for Change is the pay system implemented in the NHS in 2004. It is supported by the knowledge and skills framework which provides:

> A means of recognising the skills and knowledge that a person needs to apply to be effective in a particular NHS post. The framework will be applicable across the range of posts in the NHS ensuring better links between education and development and career and pay progression.

(DH, 2004)

Creating and sustaining a learning environment

The aims of the knowledge and skills framework are that all staff will:

- have clear and consistent development objectives
- be helped to develop in such a way that they can apply the knowledge and skills appropriate to their job
- be helped to identify and develop knowledge and skills that will support their career progression and encourage lifelong learning.

(DH, op. cit.)

Methods of creating a learning culture

**Creating
a learning
culture**

The definition of culture used in the Bristol Inquiry was:

Those attitudes, assumptions and values which condition the way in which individuals and the organisation work.

(DH, 2001a)

The report also acknowledges that organisational culture is highly complex and can be hard to change. However, as the leader of your team you can influence the culture of your area and bring about change.

Culture is not amorphous, nor immutable; we are not powerless to change it. It is in some respects no more than the sum of the actions and attitudes of many individuals.

Thus, if in some crucial areas of practice we can change the rules, the regulations and incentives, behaviour and, ultimately, attitudes will follow.

(Leape cited in DH, 2001)

Effective teams can act as a buffer against the organisational culture (Borrill *et al.*, 2001). If you are unhappy with the culture at your workplace, you can to some extent protect your team by creating a positive environment within your own area. Working cultures tend to develop because teams have learned that certain ways of working have been relatively successful in resolving problems, at least in the short term.

Problems are commonly resolved by 'fire fighting' or 'first order change'. First order change is doing more or less of something that you are already doing, rather than doing something completely new (Bergquist, 1993). For example, if you have a shortage of staff a first order change would be to book more agency nurses or recruit more staff, rather than look at why you are short of staff, which may be due to anything from poor working practices to sickness. Booking temporary staff resolves the problem on a short-term basis and delays the need to look at the real cause of the problem.

The culture within the NHS has developed since its inception in the 1940s and is set in a background of high public, patient and staff expectations but within a system of limited resources. This in turn influences the culture in the workplace and in education. Healthcare professionals are taught to deliver the best care but then work in a culture where 'getting by' is seen as a success (DH, 2001). Unfortunately, fire fighting and 'getting by' can be the block to developing a learning culture because you don't have time to integrate learning into everyday work.

It is not uncommon for teams to be working in a blame culture, where people will not admit to mistakes for fear of punishment. It is not an environment that encourages learning. Errors by definition are unintentional, but the disciplinary process and the legal system need blame to be apportioned (Runcimann & Merry, 2003). Intentional harm clearly should be punished but if an error was made by someone with good intentions, apportioning that blame can be counter-productive. What is more constructive – appropriate blame or a just culture? The questionnaire in Appendix 2 will help you to see whether you need to change the culture in your team.

If you do, in order to change that culture you will need to put the patient at the centre of your service. And to create openness you will need to involve both patients and the public in your decision making (see Chapter 8).

You will need to look at how you can enable team members to learn and implement mechanisms to support new procedures such as appraisals and mentorship. You should also consider the effectiveness of your current systems such as handover and meetings.

To develop a successful team you will need to be able to resolve any problems or challenges that the team encounters. You will need to have the skills to implement second order change (see Chapter 6), rather than simply fire fighting. Learning should be in line with the organisation's, and therefore your team's, objectives.

Creating and sustaining a learning environment

Learning styles

Learning styles

Adults learn in different ways to children. They learn best when:

- they feel secure and try things out in safety
- their needs are being met in ways that they can see are relevant and appropriate
- they know what they have to do, especially when they have been involved in setting those goals themselves
- they are actively involved and engaged
- they know how well they are doing
- they appreciate that they are welcomed and respected, both as adults and as individuals.

Deming (1989) developed the PDSA cycle based on the work of Walter Shewart. The learning cycle is a continuous circle of development. It stands for Plan, Do, Study, Act. We plan an activity and do it to the best of our ability and knowledge. We then study the outcomes and look for what we can do differently. Finally, we decide how we can do the task better and act by adjusting our methods accordingly.

Similarly, different individuals learn in different ways. Honey and Mumford (1982) describe four different types of adult learner:

the pragmatist (plan)

He/she like to try things out; they prefer to do rather than to watch. They are good at problem solving and getting things done. They like to link theory and practice and like to try the theories out.

the activist (do)

He or she will try anything once. They enjoy new experiences and challenges. They act first and consider the consequences later, they like unstructured situations and thrive on group work and discussions or debates.

the reflector (study)

He or she likes to think things through. They prefer understanding to practical application. Generally he/she will be creative and good at seeing the implications for actions.

the theorist (act)

This person prefers an organised approach to learning. They are questioning and analytical. They enjoy complex problems and like to make links with theories and models.

Most individuals will not fall into one category but will have strengths and weaknesses in each area. In order to increase learning, individuals should be encouraged to try different approaches. These characteristics can be linked to the learning cycle (see Figure 4.1). To enable you to establish team members' learning styles you can use the 'learning styles questionnaire' at www.peterhoney.com.

Figure 4.1   **The learning cycle**

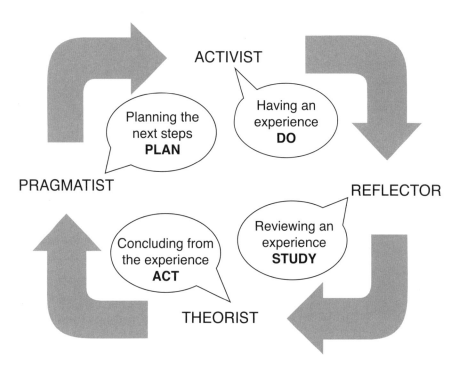

Work undertaken by the National Training Laboratory (www.ntl.org) shows that the most effective way of learning is a combination of one-to-one teaching and learning by doing. The knowledge gained this way is retained for longer. Although nurses do value attending courses and conference, the worst method of learning is sitting in lectures and seminars. Not only is it inefficient, but it is also extremely expensive in terms of time at work lost.

To enable team members to maximise their learning potential you will need to provide a variety of learning opportunities. Ideally, these opportunities should be part of the usual working day.

Appraisals

Appraisals

Performance appraisals are an important part of effective management and evaluation of your team members. In spite of the Department of Health (DH) asking trusts to report the percentage of staff undertaking formal appraisals and widespread recognition of their value, a recent Healthcare Commission survey of NHS staff found that more than 33% of staff have never been appraised (Healthcare Commission, 2004).

The purpose of appraisals is to:

- support individual development and identify training needs
- improve team performance
- feed into business planning
- agree objectives
- monitor and maintain standards.

Appraisals support the implementation of a learning culture because they provide the evidence that all staff have equal access to training and development and are encouraged to develop new skills. An appraisal helps to identify development needs and the appropriate method of learning for each member of staff.

There is a problem, however, that there is a common belief that appraisals can be used to motivate employees by using 'carrots and sticks' or rewards and punishment. This is based on the premise that people are only motivated through incentives and disincentives, but studies into why nurses stay in jobs show that this is not the case. In order to make appraisals effective they need to be based on individual development and progress, and they must be based on fact.

Performance appraisal is one tool that you can use to manage the performance of staff but it should not be the only one that you use. Appraisals should be used to review past performance and plan for the future. They should be an opportunity for discussion where the appraisee contributes as much as the appraiser.

Conducting an appraisal

Conducting an appraisal

Your hospital will have a policy relating to appraisals and this will include templates and a structure for the sessions as well as the training needs for those undertaking appraisals. The training will incorporate questioning and listening skills and giving and receiving feedback.

The process of appraisal consists of four basic stages:

Measurement – individual performance should be measured against objectives set at the previous appraisal or at induction. This will include a self-assessment and management assessment against the relevant knowledge and skills framework.

Feedback – all feedback should be constructive, honest and non-judgemental to enable the individual to improve their work.

Discussion – discussion should focus on the support that the individual needs and be based on the knowledge and skills framework, including any requirements for training and development.

Agreement – both the appraisee and appraiser must agree to any actions or objectives set during the appraisal.

The appraisal should relate to the Knowledge and Skills Framework (DH, 2004) and include the development review process. Your organisation will have policies and procedures to help you with this. You can also refer to your human resources department for further advice.

The development review process consists of:

reviewing how individuals are applying their knowledge and skills in their current post and identifying whether they have any development needs

developing a Personal Development Plan detailing the learning and development required

evaluating the learning and development and reflecting on how it has been applied in their role.

(DH, 2004)

It should therefore be an inherent part of the appraisal process. The DH provides templates for the development review process on its website.

Before undertaking an appraisal you should organise a date, time and venue. This sounds obvious but lack of preparation will mean that the session will be rushed and neither of you will be in the right mood to get the most from it.

The appraisee should be given plenty of notice and advised to prepare for the session. They need to think about the progress they have made, the training they have undertaken and the support they have needed. They will also need to consider what they want to achieve in the coming year and how they hope to do it. It is good practice for the appraisee to bring this information in written form as this will help them to remember everything they want to discuss. However, don't make this too onerous as some people will find it intimidating.

The venue should be quiet and without interruptions. This can be difficult to achieve in a busy ward environment but it is essential so that the appraisal can focus solely on the individual and is completely confidential. Avoid cancelling an appraisal, where possible, as this undermines the importance of the session and the preparation the individual has made. Again, this can be difficult in a clinical environment, but it is essential that appraisals are seen as a high priority.

You will need to have the appraisee's job description, details of the training and development they have had and records of previous appraisals. You should consider the points that you wish to discuss with the individual prior to the meeting, including measurement and feedback.

Questioning skills

Questioning skills

The purpose of questioning is to obtain information. In an appraisal you will need to ask the right questions to get the information you want.

Use **open-ended** questions which invite an actual explanation for a response. Questions that begin with 'how', 'what' and 'why' are typical. Reflecting questions enable you to clarify what has been said and get the individual talking freely and in depth. Reflecting questions encourage 'active listening', using the appraisee's words to draw out further information. They often begin:

'You said that...'

'You sound as if...'

'I get the feeling that...'

You will also need to use extending questions to invite further explanation and to prompt a further answer:

'How else could...?'

'Could you tell me more about...?'

Comparative questions are also useful for getting the appraisee to evaluate one situation against another:

'What has it been like since...?'

'What difference has...'

Keep notes throughout the session. It is useful to summarise what has been said at the end, using statements of the form:

'These seem to be the key points you have expressed...'

Listen carefully throughout and put the information into a logical order.

Listening skills

Listening skills

According to Mehrabian and Ferris (1967) when we are communicating face to face with people we pay most of our attention to body language and voice tone and only seven per cent of our attention is on what people actually say. The way you listen is important, but what you hear may not be just about what is being said.

If you interrupt the speaker or are easily distracted, the speaker will get the impression that you're not interested in what they are saying, even if you are.

Don't jump to conclusions. Many people stop listening to a speaker when they think they have the gist of the conversation or know what they are trying to say next. If you are not sure of what the speaker is saying, ask:

'Do you mean...?' or

'Did I understand you to say...?'

Don't let yourself be distracted by the environment or by the speaker's appearance, accent, mannerisms, or word use. Paying too much attention to these can break your concentration and make you miss the point of the conversation.

Make eye contact with the speaker. Show them you understand what they are saying by nodding your head, maintaining an upright posture, and, if appropriate, interjecting an occasional comment.

Giving feedback

Giving feedback

There are several models for giving feedback; one is the EEC framework (also referred to as Facts, Feelings and Future) which is simple and easy to remember.

Example (Facts)

Tell the person what they did.

Give the facts and be specific.

Effect (Feelings)

Tell them the effect their action had and any impact it had on people's feelings, positive and negative.

Change (Future)

Encourage the person to come up with ideas on how they could develop further.

To be useful, feedback requires the giver to feel concern for the person receiving feedback and want to help, rather than hurt, the other person. It is important to focus on what you are doing as you give feedback. This helps you to engage in a two-way exchange with some depth of communication.

Feedback is most effective when the receiver has invited comment or is prepared to receive it; this is one good reason to plan appraisals in advance. It gives the appraisee an opportunity to identify and explore particular areas of concern.

Successful feedback is specific and deals clearly with particular incidents and behaviour. If you wish to give judgements, you must state clearly that these are subjective and let the person concerned make an evaluation.

The most useful feedback is focused on behaviour that can be changed by the appraisee. This will form part of their objectives for the coming year.

Review

Review

The most common timing for appraisals is once a year, however you may want to undertake a review more frequently, perhaps every three to six months. This could be a shorter session where the objectives are reviewed to check that the individual is on course and doesn't need any additional support or training. This may seem time consuming but it can make an end-of-year appraisal more manageable and it is less likely that there will be any surprises.

Career development

Career development

Career planning is a continuous process of self-assessment and goal planning.

(ICN, 2001)

Helping your team to develop their careers is an important part of the line manager's role and an important part of the appraisal process. It has been shown to be a useful incentive (Buchan *et al.*, 2000; McCarty, 2002) and it also encourages staff retention and reduces turnover.

The responsibility for career planning should be placed with the employee but they will require support from the line manager in identifying potential options, training opportunities and the possibilities for flexible working and secondments. It may help to involve someone from your human resources department to give another perspective on what is available.

Employees should be encouraged to think about the climate they work in, the potential changes nationally, professionally and locally. They should consider what they like and dislike and what their values are. Encourage them to get a mentor and to read professional journals and national newspapers. Looking at adverts for jobs not related to their current area of practice, and even outside the healthcare environment, will help them identify what attracts them to some jobs and not to others.

Often an obstacle to career development is that individuals are reluctant to take a sideways move but such a move can often allow the individual to develop further before making a move up the ladder.

Make sure that you always advertise posts internally as well as externally and that you share secondment opportunities with the whole team.

Don't focus career development just on senior members of the team. Consider succession planning; how will you replace key members of your team if they leave? Allowing people to 'act up' into roles is really good development if the individual is ready for the additional responsibility. Be careful not to raise expectations, however. Allowing someone to act up sometimes leads to the assumption that that person will get the job if it becomes available.

Mentorship

Mentoring has a long history, the terminology originating from Homer's Odyssey. Mentor was a friend of Odysseus who brought up his son, Telemachus, while he was away. The term originally became commonplace in traditionally male professions such as medicine and law. It became part of nursing terminology in the 1980s when it was mainly associated with those undertaking formal learning programmes either as a pre- or post-registration nurse. More recently it has been adopted throughout the profession.

There are a number of definitions of mentoring. The Standing Committee on Postgraduate Medical & Dental Education (SCOPME) has defined mentoring as:

> *a process whereby an experienced, highly regarded, empathetic person (the mentor) guides another individual in the development and re-examination of their own ideas, learning and personal and professional development.*

(SCOPME, 1998)

Kay and Hinds describe mentoring as:

> *a relationship between two parties, who are not connected within a line management structure, in which one party (the mentor) guides the other (the mentee) through a period of change and towards an agreed objective.*

(Kay and Hinds, 2002)

Byrne and Keefe's definition of 'mentor' is widely accepted:

> *a person who helps a more junior person develop professionally through a combination of advising on projects, skills development, creation of opportunities, and personal growth in an intense manner over an extended period of time.*

(Byrne and Keefe, 2002)

The combination of these definitions describes mentoring very well. Mentoring is a process between two people over a period of time, there is no set time frame for mentoring but at the outset an agreement should be made between both parties about when and how to end the relationship.

The mentor is a person who is more experienced, respected and more senior than the mentee. They are not however, in a line management position with the mentee. This is important because a line manager is not in an objective position and therefore cannot fulfil the true role of a mentor.

The role of the mentor is to help the personal and professional development of the mentee, by supporting them to re-examine their ideas and actions. The mentor will advise and guide, rather than tell the mentee what to do. They will help the mentee meet an agreed set of objectives made at the start of the sessions.

Importantly, the mentor will also create learning opportunities for the mentee. Nurses often tell me that they use their colleague or friend as a mentor. There is nothing at all wrong with using colleagues and friends as support, but it is unlikely that they will be able to fulfil the true role of the mentor, particularly when it comes to creating learning opportunities.

Benefits of mentoring

Mentoring is one of the most cost-effective ways of developing people within your team (Clutterbuck, 2004) and it also has a number of other benefits. Maddison undertook a study of nurse managers in California and identified a number of benefits of mentoring including: increased thinking skills, raised self esteem, increased job satisfaction and commitment to the role, a higher level of political awareness and increased performance (Maddison, 1994). Yoder also found that nurses with a mentor were likely to stay longer in their jobs (Yoder, 1995).

There is further evidence to support that having a mentor will help share nursing values, standards and culture as well as increasing clinical competence (Smith *et al.*, 2002). Mentoring is therefore a useful way of implementing a learning culture within your team.

Finding a mentor

If you want to implement mentorship in your area, start by getting yourself a mentor. Once you understand the benefits on a personal level and have developed your confidence you will more easily be able to act as a mentor yourself. Your line manager may be able to help you find a suitable person. Don't be afraid to ask someone to be your mentor even if you perceive them to be either too senior or too busy. They will be flattered to be asked and the worst they can do is say 'no'. The best mentor will be challenging so don't ask someone who is a friend or close colleague. You need someone who will give you opportunities that you wouldn't otherwise have.

Role modelling

Role modelling

A role model is defined by the Oxford English Dictionary (2005) as:

> *'someone who, in the performance of a role is taken as a model by others'.*

Role modelling has always been used as a form of teaching in nursing as it is a method of teaching by example. It is a method by which individuals learn professional behaviour. A mentor may sometimes act as a role model, but a role model does not have to be a mentor. In fact, during our work we continually act as a role model although it may be unintentionally at times.

The characteristics of a good role model are that they are clinically competent, have good communication skills and are enthusiastic about their role. There are also poor role models who may adversely affect the individual's development. Role modelling is a really powerful way of learning but we should be aware of the impact of negative role modelling.

You can only role model if you and senior members of your team are working alongside more junior staff. Evidence shows that where there are more qualified nurses working clinically the standards of care are better (West *et al.*, 2004). This is partly because of the power of role modelling.

If you want your team members to learn good practices and professional behaviour you should be conscious of yourself as a role model and make sure that other people in your team are too.

Shadowing

Shadowing

Shadowing is an excellent way for people to find what is involved in other roles. It is a really good way of encouraging individuals to get a broader perspective and helping team members understand each other's roles and responsibilities.

Encourage members of your team to shadow yourself or other people within the multi-disciplinary team. Make sure that they think about the purpose of the shadowing and draft out a list of aims and objectives before the event. Then ask them to discuss these with the person they are shadowing. At the end of the experience they should discuss what happened with the person they are shadowing and identify what they have learnt. Both parties should agree to confidentiality at the beginning as they may be exposed to sensitive situations.

Handover

Handover

Most clinical teams use a form of handover to pass patient information from one shift to another. Most of the articles written about handover support the need for walk round handover (Kelly, 2005; Watkins, 1993; McMahon, 1990). The benefits of walk round handover are that it is patient-centred, it tends to be quicker and it enables the patient to ask questions, particularly when coupled with electronic nursing handover sheets which increase the information that can be shared and reduce the time spent passing on 'routine' details such as name, consultant and age. The research shows that nurses can spend varying amounts of time at handover. Making the handover more patient-centred will mean that you can involve the patient more in their care and use the time to educate both them and the staff. This doesn't have to happen every time with every patient, but utilising this time effectively will help the team get used to the idea that learning is part of everyday working practices.

Meetings

Meetings

Running effective meetings will be discussed further in Chapter 7. Like handover, meetings should be used as a learning opportunity. The tone of the meeting will impact not only on attendance but on the prospect of attendees learning from the discussions. The chair of the meeting should encourage openness and learning by encouraging questions and contributions from everyone. Items not resolved within the meeting should be carried over to the next agenda and the attendees encouraged to resolve the issue (by reading articles, asking other members of the team and so on).

Try and make sure that all team members have an opportunity to attend. Buddy up with another ward to provide staff cover while the meeting is taking place.

Other methods of learning in practice

Learning in practice

You may already use a variety of methods of learning in your environment. Here are some that you might wish to think about.

Ward rounds

Ward rounds have traditionally been a part of teaching for junior doctors and medical students. It has been accepted practice that the ward leader attends the ward rounds but why not encourage more junior members to attend as a learning opportunity.

Multi-disciplinary team meetings

These are an ideal opportunity for learning. Try and make sure that everyone gets an opportunity to attend.

Poster displays

On its own, reading is not an effective way to get people to retain knowledge but using posters as a reminder is a cheap and cheerful way of sharing information. Why not ask staff who have completed projects or dissertations as part of a course to share their learning via a poster?

Quizzes

Take it in turns to write a quiz and offer a small prize (sweets, a pen or similar) to the person with the most correct answers.

Conclusion

Creating a learning environment is an essential component of improving patient outcomes and staff working conditions. The factors that promote learning are adequate staffing levels (see Chapter 1), a system of mentoring, effective communication, individual appraisals and clear clinical governance policies (see also Chapter 4). The most efficient methods of learning are one-to-one teaching and learning by doing, so effective role modelling will not only help you to share your values but also improve your team's clinical skills.

You will need to be creative about incorporating learning into everyday practice, but it can be done with few resources.

Chapter 5
Performance management

Werner and DeSimone define performance management as: '*simply a matter of expecting tasks to be done on time*' (Werner and DeSimone, 2005). Unfortunately, it is anything but simple and can be a legal minefield and is therefore one of the things that managers do less well. Managing good performance is relatively simple, while managing poor performance is not, but the process of performance management should always be as positive as possible.

Christine Beasley, Chief Nursing Officer for England, says that:

> *healthcare in England benefits enormously from having a dedicated, committed and highly skilled workforce, focused on offering quality care for patients. However, sometimes things go awry and a healthcare professional may find their practice called into question.*
>
> (DH, 2006)

People who are not performing well need to be supported appropriately to improve their performance for their own benefit, for the good of patients and to help the team.

Strebler defines poor performance as when: '*an employee's behaviour or performance might fall below the required standard*' (Strebler, 2004). This might include poor attitude, constantly failing to meet personal objectives or an inability to cope with their workload.

Your organisation's human resource department will be able to offer advice and support in dealing with persistent poor performers. *Handling Concerns about the Performance of Healthcare Professionals: Principles of Good Practice* (DH, 2006) outlines the principles for handling performance concerns and is a useful resource.

Performance management is a key part of a line manager's role and there are some basic principles that you should have in place. The process of performance management comprises:

standards and goal setting – so that individuals know what is expected of them

coaching – ensuring that individuals are supported to develop and meet the expectations of the team and organisation

rewards – giving praise and rewarding good performance

individual development – ensuring individuals have the skills to deliver what is expected of them.

The CIPD 'Performance Management Survey Report' (CIPD, 2005a) shows that performance management works best when it is an integrated part of management, linked to quantifiable measures (see Chapter 9) and a continuous process rather than a one-off event.

Performance management starts from the moment that someone commences their employment, at which point your expectations of them should be clearly outlined. These will include mandatory expectations (employment contracts, policies and procedures) with which the employee has to comply. Part of their induction should include an introduction to the relevant policies and procedures (for example those relating to time off work, bullying and harassment, personal appearance, time keeping and smoking) and the contract of employment along with an explanation and a check that the individual understands the content and the implications for them. By law (the Employment Act 2002) all employees must also be given a written statement of the dismissal, disciplinary and grievance procedures for your organisation. This is followed by some basic expectations which will form the job description. This will outline what their individual role is.

Standards and goal-setting

Standards & goal-setting

The standards and levels of performance required must be known and understood by the employee. They will be related to the appropriate knowledge and skills framework. Most importantly this should be documented in their personal file. These standards and levels of performance provide a benchmark against which performance can be evaluated.

Setting standards for performance and behaviour forms an important part of developing a learning culture (see Chapter 4). Goal setting will take place at the appraisal or performance development review (see Chapter 5). These should be related to the knowledge and skills framework outline for the post. These must be agreed with the employee and recorded in writing.

Coaching

Coaching

As an employer you have a responsibility to ensure that employees perform effectively. The Nursing and Midwifery Council (NMC, 2004) outlines the following responsibilities of employers:

- employees should be recruited with the skills to undertake the work they are employed to do
- they should have a full induction to their area of work
- training and supervision should be provided
- provision should be made for preceptorship and mentoring
- clinical supervision should be available
- employees should receive regular performance appraisals (at least annually)

Just as the employer has responsibilities, so does the registered nurse. The NMC Code of Professional Conduct (2002) clearly states that the individual practitioner must maintain knowledge and competence, keep up-to-date, be able to practice competently without direct supervision and acknowledge any limits to their competence.

Individual development

Individual development

The employer does have a duty to ensure that the employee is in a position to carry out the job – that there are no obstacles preventing them from carrying out a task and that they have the skills and competence to do it. So what do you do if a member of your team is not performing well?

Firstly, you must identify the problem. This could be anything from working too slowly to harassment, abuse and stealing. The nature of the problem will determine your approach. Your organisation will have a disciplinary policy which will outline how you must deal with matters of misconduct. There will also be an absence policy which will set out the procedure for dealing with staff who have had time off work and a capability policy about dealing with an individual's lack of capability to do their job.

You need to be clear what your expectations are and in what way the individual is failing to meet them. (Using the knowledge and skills framework will help you be clear about the problem.) Then you need to decide whether the problem is worth tackling. If the problem is serious then you need to act quickly; patient safety must be of greatest importance. Involve your human resources manager and your line manager.

Failing to tackle even a minor problem may not be the best solution as poor performance can have an impact on motivation and retention as well as efficiency (Strebler, 2004). It also means that you are not giving an individual an opportunity to rectify the problem. Early intervention may resolve the issue by bringing it to their attention. An informal approach is usually a good start. If this doesn't work you can follow it up with a more formal method.

Make sure that any communication with the employee is clear. Describe the behaviour that is causing the problem and provide evidence. Try and find out why they are acting in the way that they are. Describe the impact of their behaviour and how it is making you or other individuals feel. Finally, explore the options for the future and how you can both rectify the problem. Make sure that you record the discussion and put in writing to the individual what you have discussed. You may need to provide extra supervision or training, a checklist to help them prioritise what they need to do or an action plan with clear objectives and timescales.

Don't forget to give frequent feedback (see Chapter 4) and make sure that it is positive if they are performing well. Establish some timescales within which the individual must make the changes and make sure that they agree that they are realistic. Strebler uses the acronym 'TAPS' for dealing with performance issues.

*Feedback should be **T**imely and early*

*You should use an **A**ppropriate management style and response*

*Keep it **P**rivate*

*Make it **S**pecific to performance and make sure it is factual.*

(Strebler, 2004)

As always, remember to document what has been agreed. You should include:

● what the unsatisfactory performance was

● what your expectations are

● the timescales

● what will happen if the expectations are not met.

If an informal approach fails to work you may need to take a formal approach (see 'Making it formal' later in this chapter).

Rewards and recognition

Rewards and recognition

Performance management is linked to reward and recognition. Recognition has been shown to be important for nurse morale (Cronin, 1999; Hader, 2004). Rewards and recognition are important motivating factors and therefore can increase performance. Rewards and recognition do not have to be financially based; in fact, in the current financial climate it is unrealistic to think of rewards in terms of money.

There are a number of non-monetary awards that you can give and these are listed below.

Examples of non-monetary rewards and recognition

● Saying 'thank you'

● Giving praise, privately

● Formal public recognition, such as award ceremonies

● Giving praise in front of peers

● Letters of appreciation – particularly from a more senior manager (matron, nursing director)

● Copying cards from patients which name particular nurses to those named and senior nurses

- Recognition in the hospital newsletter
- Selection to represent the manager at a special meeting (of interest to the employee)
- Selection for a particular role, such as link nurse
- Invitation to attend events as an observer
- Opportunity for more responsibility
- Positive cards for patients and/or staff to give to nurses whom they think have performed well; the nurse collects the cards to give to the ward leader. The ward leader then recognises the nurse using one of the above methods
- Awarding employee of the month (define how this can be achieved first)
- Recognising people's birthdays, either from the team or from yourself as line manager
- Recommending an employee to speak at a conference
- Nomination to national nurse of the year awards (www.nursing-standard.co.uk).

Recognition should be given to people who have demonstrated that they have learnt from mistakes as well as to those who have made an achievement. In that way you will help to create a learning culture.

The key to giving recognition is that it should be genuine and sincere. It should also be fair. No matter how small the recognition, members of the team may take it very seriously. As line manager to a team I once started an 'Employee of the Month' award. It started as a light-hearted event and the person who won was given a certificate and a prize. The prize could be worth no more than £2 (I brought it out of my own money!) but I was amazed at how seriously the team took it and how well it worked in terms of motivating people. Naturally, it didn't work for everyone and that's the key to recognition and reward – you have to use different methods for different people.

Rewards and recognition do not necessarily have to be given just to individuals; you might also want to consider team rewards. The team should be involved in developing the reward system and the measures that you will use. The disadvantages to team rewards are that it may not acknowledge individual effort. It may also result in the team performing just enough to achieve the minimum result. Nonetheless, the benefits are that it can help build the team and encourage poor performers to improve their standards to that of other team members.

Measuring team performance

Tools for Measuring Team Performance

Team Collaboration Index – Aram, Morgan and Esbeck, 1971

Team Anomie Scale – Farrell, Heinemann and Schmitt, 1992

Group Development Assessment – Jones and Bearley, 1993

Team Development Rating Scale – Kormanski and Mozenter, 1987

Analysing Team Effectiveness – McGregor, Bennis and McGregor, 1967

Team Assessment Worksheets – McClane, 1992

(ICN, 2005)

What factors affect performance?

Factors affecting performance

There may be a legitimate reason why someone is performing poorly and this might be relatively easy to overcome, avoiding the need to progress to the formal procedure. It might include lack of motivation, lack of feedback, no goal clarity and a lack of training and development. Other factors can be poor health or domestic problems, inappropriate delegation and shift working and long hours.

Poor health or domestic problems

It may be helpful to refer an individual who is having problems outside of work to your occupational health department where they will offer confidential support and advice to the member of staff and advise you as line manager on the best ways to manage the situation.

Inappropriate delegation

Delegation is essential in the workplace. Without it the work simply would not get done. Delegation helps to develop staff and to ensure that the workload is distributed and completed in a timely manner. But poor delegation can lead to poor performance due to overload or an inability of the individual to complete the task.

To avoid this situation make sure that the individual has the skills required to undertake the task. Help them to prioritise by explaining to them the importance of the task in relation to the other things they are expected to do. Give them a time in which to complete the task and make sure you give them the opportunity to seek help if they need it.

You should be aware of everyone's strengths and weaknesses in your team. You do not always need to play to people's strengths. A person's weakness may be seen as a development opportunity, as long as you can ensure that they have the support and supervision to undertake the task and further develop their skills. Take into account their maturity and relevant experience. Consider their workload and what they will get out of the task.

Be aware that, as a registered nurse, you remain accountable for tasks that you delegate. The NMC says:

> You may be expected to delegate care delivery to others who are not registered nurses or midwives. Such delegation must not compromise existing care but must be directed to meeting the needs and serving the interests of patients and clients. You remain accountable for the appropriateness of the delegation, for ensuring that the person who does the work is able to do it and that adequate supervision or support is provided.

> (Clause 4.6 of the NMC Code of Professional Conduct)

As a practitioner registered with the NMC, you are responsible for ensuring that those to whom responsibilities are delegated are competent. You must assess this competence and determine what preparation unqualified and registered staff need.

Shift working and long hours

Around 60% of nurses work shifts (RCN, 2002). This is unavoidable when providing a 24 hour service seven days a week. The consequences of working shifts include lack of sleep, poor eating patterns and mental and physical health problems (Fitzpatrick, 1999; ICN, 2000; Wilson, 2002) which can lead to poor performance. Although 43% of nurses say that they don't like the shifts they work, and 56% say they cannot self roster, the evidence is that where nurses choose their own shifts or self roster there is increased morale and job satisfaction and the effects of shift working are less (Edell-Gustafsson, 2002).

The Royal College of Nursing (RCN) has said that:

> All nurses should have the opportunity and ability to review their

own work patterns and to secure the working arrangements which best suit their professional and personal interests and their commitment to patients' care.

(RCN, 1997)

The length of the working week and shifts also affect safety. Research has shown that working more than 40 hours a week significantly increases the risk of making an error. Working more than eight and half hours per day also increases that risk (Rogers *et al.*, 2004).

The European Working Time Directive, enacted in UK law as the Working Time Regulations with effect from 1 October 1998, is mandatory and restricts working hours. Employees should work no more than 48 hours a week (over a reference period) and should have 11 hours of continuous rest in 24 hours. Night workers should work no more than eight hours in 24 hours (over a reference period). This is supported by the DH's Improving Working Lives initiative (DH, 2004a).

If you identify poor performance in someone and they identify shift working as the cause you should try to offer them support and look at ways of making their shift working more manageable. This can be quite difficult when you are trying to please all the members of your team but there are some things that you can put in place which will help the whole team

Reducing the impact of shift working

Options for reducing the impact of shift working

- Self rostering
- Making off duty available to staff in advance to allow individuals to forward plan
- Forward rotation (clockwise) (earlies followed by lates followed by nights)
- Allowing staff to choose the number of nights they work in a row
- A minimum of two days off together
- Night and evening shifts should be shorter than day shifts
- Computerised rostering
- Individualised rostering

(ICN, 2000; Wilson, 2002)

Making it formal

Making it formal

If an individual continues to perform inadequately following an informal approach you may consider making it more formal. It is extremely important that you consult your human resources department and line manager before proceeding with a formal approach as failure to follow the procedure could lead to an appeal by the individual.

Disciplinary and grievance procedures are covered by the Employment Act 2002. It sets out the minimum requirements for dealing with disciplinary issues. Your organisation's policies and procedures will reflect this and may expect you to do more than is described here.

There are two main categories of behaviour that can lead to a disciplinary process – poor performance or misconduct. The process for poor performance is slightly different to that of misconduct. Described here is the process for poor performance.

The first step is to write to the employee to inform them that the process is being taken further. You must advise them that the letter will be followed by a meeting. The time between the letter and the meeting should be long enough to allow the employee to prepare. The employee should be sent copies of any documents that will be used at the meeting. The Advisory Conciliation and Arbitration Service (ACAS) provides advice on its website about whether employees can be accompanied to this and any subsequent meetings at www.acas.org.uk. The meeting should be held at a time that is acceptable to the employee and employer. The employee will also be entitled to bring someone along to the meeting for support.

At the meeting the employer explains the issue and the supporting evidence. The employee is given opportunity to explain their case and to present supporting evidence too. They are also given the opportunity to ask questions.

Following the meeting the employer makes a decision as to whether this will be followed by the disciplinary procedure. The employee should be informed in writing as soon as possible as to what the decision is, even if the decision is to do nothing more. It is good practice to give the employee another chance at this stage and so you can again clarify the problem, set out your expectations and timescales and give them a review date. You should also be clear about the support you will give to them to help them improve. Make sure that everything is recorded. The employee should also be advised that if they do not improve at this stage they may be given a final written warning.

A final written warning will outline the issue and what will happen if there is still no improvement. It will also set out their rights of appeal. The warning should be kept in their personal file for 12 months, after which time it should be removed.

The options following an unsuccessful final written warning depend on the terms and conditions of the employment contract and your organisational policies. The employee may be demoted or dismissed. The decision making should not be your responsibility as immediate line manager.

This process will apply to both qualified and unqualified nurses. For qualified nurses you will need to consider when to involve the NMC.

Reporting to the NMC

Reporting to the Nursing and Midwifery Council

The role of the NMC is to protect the public and take action if a registrant fails to maintain the standards set for entry to the register. Anyone can make an allegation of unfitness to practice due to either misconduct or lack of competence. You should only refer to the NMC if you consider the employee will not make any further improvement.

Lack of competence is defined by the NMC as:

> *Lack of knowledge, skill or judgement of such nature that the registrant is unfit to practice safely and effectively in any field which the registrant claims to be competent or seeks to practice.*

(NMC, 2004)

The NMC will not usually become involved until you have already attempted to manage the situation yourself. If you have followed the basic principles of good management as outlined in this chapter and have documented each stage of the process then you can make a referral to the NMC.

The NMC will ask for all supporting evidence in relation to your complaint. This will be submitted to the Investigating Committee who will decide whether the case is misconduct or lack of competence. Examples of misconduct include physical and verbal abuse, theft, deliberate failure to deliver adequate care and deliberate failure to keep proper records. The Investigating Committee will inform the registrant who will then receive copies of the documentation and be asked to submit a written response to the panel. The Committee will then decide whether there is a case to answer. To put it into perspective, in 2004–5 only two cases were referred to the Lack of Competence Committee (NMC, 2005). If the complaint is substantiated the NMC has four options:

- a striking off order (the registrant is removed from the register)

- a suspension order

- a conditions of practice order

- a caution order.

A registrant can only receive a striking off order for lack of competence if they have had two years' continuous suspension or conditions of practice order.

If you consider that the case justifies an immediate interim suspension from the register (before an NMC hearing) you should contact the NMC immediately. This might be appropriate when the police have become involved in the case, for example. The NMC contact details can be found on their website (www.nmc-org.uk).

It is important to recognise that dismissal from employment does not necessarily mean that an employee will be removed from the NMC register. It is a completely separate process.

Avoiding discrimination

Avoiding discrimination

The law prevents people and organisations from discriminating against particular groups. The legislation includes:

- Equal Pay Act 1970

- Sex Discrimination Act 1975

- Race Relations Act 1976

- Disability Discrimination Act 1995

- Employment Rights Act 1996

- Race Relations Act 2000

- Employment Act 2002

- Race Relations Act 1976 (Amendment) Regulations 2003

- Religion or Belief Regulations 2003

- Sexual Orientation Regulations 2003

- Age Discrimination Regulations 2006
- Part Time Workers Regulations 2000
- Fixed Term Employee Regulations 2002

This legislation applies not only when you are employing staff but to existing staff too. It therefore impacts on terms of employment, opportunities for promotion, training, secondments and reward and recognition. It also applies to the disciplinary process and dismissal (ACAS, 2004).

The British Medical Association (BMA) defines the different types of discrimination in this way:

> **direct discrimination** – when an individual has been treated less favourably than others in similar circumstances
>
> **indirect discrimination** – where some people are less likely to be able to comply/fulfil a requirement or criterion than others
>
> **victimisation** – if an individual has been treated less favourably because they have complained about discrimination or supported someone else who has
>
> **harassment** – any conduct or comment, which is unreasonable, unwelcome or offensive and causes the recipient to feel threatened, humiliated or embarrassed
>
> **bullying** – misuse of power or position. Bullying behaviour criticises, condemns and humiliates people and can undermine their ability and confidence.

(BMA, 2004)

NMC code of conduct

The NMC Code of Professional Conduct states that:

> *You are expected to work co-operatively within teams and to respect the skills, expertise and contributions of your colleagues. You must treat them fairly and without discrimination.*
>
> *Your organization will have an equal opportunities and harassment policy which you should be familiar with. To help you avoid discrimination you should ensure that every member of your team has an appraisal and personal development plan (see Chapters 4 and 5). Advertise all your vacancies, even if only internally, and respond quickly to any complaints that members of the team make about discrimination. Make sure you and all of your team members have equal opportunities training. Seek advice from your human resources department if you are in any doubt.*

How do you know whether you're getting it right?

The CIPD surveyed managers and found that the following factors indicate that performance management is working:

- communication is effective
- productivity is high – in nursing this might be demonstrated in improving performance measures (see Chapter 9) or an improvement in the quality of patient care
- goals are achieved – this will be apparent in performance appraisals
- motivation is high
- regular two way feedback is taking place
- staff turnover has decreased
- skills are developed
- the workforce is happy.

(CIPD, 2005a)

Assess your team regularly to make sure that you are getting it right.

Chapter 6
Understanding change and its impact on team performance

The National Health Service is constantly changing for a number of reasons. As a publicly-funded service it will always be included in the manifestos of political parties. Many of the changes that have taken place recently are discussed in other chapters in this book. The ethos behind the current health service reforms is the desire to establish a patient-led service. This is being delivered by a number of policies including Practice Based Commissioning (DH, 2004c), Choice (DH, 2003), Patient and Public Involvement (DH, 2004b), Payment by Results (DH, 2004d) and Agenda for Change (DH, 2004e).

If you ask staff working on the 'shop floor' about changes in the NHS they are less likely to cite national policies and are more likely to talk about local changes. These may include large organisational changes that impact on them – such as redundancies – but will also include the changes in management structure, computerisation and changes in uniform and visiting times. These are the things that affect them personally.

Change can affect people in different ways but by managing change effectively the stress and anxiety to individuals can be minimised.

Why do we need to change?

There are a number of reasons for changing the way we work.

Reasons for changing

New evidence
New evidence may be produced locally, within specialisms and professions or nationally. Whatever its source, new research creates a demand for new treatments and drugs and the NHS has to find a way of funding them fairly and equitably.

Improving patient outcomes

Increasing and changing patient expectations

Public and patients have greater knowledge of what is available to them and expect a certain quality of service. This is reflected in the number and type of complaints and concerns that trusts receive on a daily basis.

New technology

Even the way we record temperature and pulses has changed enormously over the last 10 to 20 years and few of us would wish to return to the old practices. However, new technology means learning new ways of working in order to make best use of the equipment available.

The need to give value for money

The NHS is a publicly-funded service, paid for through national insurance. Chief executives are now held to account for the budgets that they hold. In 2005 and 2006 many trusts went into an overspend, which led to service cuts and job redundancies. The NHS has to provide a value-for-money service and this means adapting the way we work to make the service more efficient.

Ageing population

In 2005 the number of people aged over 85 had increased to 1.2 million and the number aged 50 and over to 20 million (DWP, 2005). In most parts of the country, older people are the biggest users of health services. The rise in the number of older people in the population will put additional demands on the health service and require healthcare workers to work differently. This may mean managing increased demands on the service or a need to work outside the acute setting as care moves more into the community (DH, 2006b).

Increasingly diverse population

According to National Statistics (www.statistics.gov.uk) in 2001 92% of the population in the UK was white, with the remaining 7.9% of the population made up from other ethnic groups. There has also been a rise in migration to the UK, mostly from the ten countries that joined the European community in 2004. This inevitably means that healthcare workers need to look at the way they work in relation to the needs of a changing population.

How does change affect people?

Effects of change

Research shows that most changes do not achieve their original objectives because of people issues and that 50% of people feel that change in their organisation is not managed well (OPP, 2004). Organisational change is a source of workplace stress and can affect physical health and increase sickness rates (Collins, 2006) and therefore morale and workload. On the other hand, change can be a motivator. It can allow people to take on different roles and responsibilities and provide them with opportunities they might not otherwise have had.

How people respond to change will depend on how the change impinges on their lives. If we choose to make a change in our lives which will have a relatively small effect we will be able to cope well with it. However, if we choose to make a change and the impact is high – such as moving house or changing jobs – we will probably cope with the change but it will still cause us some anxiety. If we have no choice about the change we will react badly to it and the severity of the reaction will depend on the effect it has on our lives.

Figure 6.1   **Impact of change**

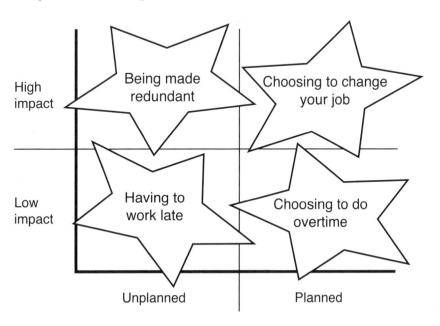

William Bridges talks about 'transition' as the way that people come to terms with change.

> *Transition* is not just a nice way to say **change**. *It is the inner process through which people come to terms with a change, as they let go of the way things used to be and reorient themselves to the way that things are now. In an organization, managing **transition** means helping people to make that difficult process less painful and disruptive.*

www.wmbridges.com

He describes the stages of transition as being similar to that of the grieving process. There are three stages of transition: endings, the neutral zone and the new beginning.

Endings

Unlike the stages of change, transition starts with an ending. This is the stage at which people have to let go. Commonly people feel a sense of loss; this might be a loss of identity, responsibility, relationships, environment, control or meaning. It makes people frightened and anxious and can often create a climate of blame.

Neutral zone

The neutral zone is a time of uncertainty and confusion. Some people will be trying to get back to the old situation and others will be striving toward the new. It can last a long time, particularly in situations such as mergers where the neutral zone can go on as long as two years (Bridges & Bridges, 2000).

Some people will continue to work in the old way for as long as the transition lasts.

New beginnings

New beginnings is when people start to explore the new situation. They need to start behaving in a new way and can feel anxious about this especially where there is a blame culture as they will be concerned about their competence and ability to perform.

Managing transitions

Managing transitions

Before you embark on any change you should be clear why you are making a change and be able to explain this succinctly and clearly to your team. Don't assume that every member of your team will understand the need to change. Make sure that you give them lots of information; different people will require different types of information.

Conceptual people

These types of people like ideas not data. They like to see the big picture and they want to be involved in deciding what needs to change and why.

Analytical people

Unlike conceptual people, this group of people like to have as much data as possible. They want to know: how many? how much? They then need to analyse this information, decide what it means and then they will make a decision.

Behavioural people

These people are relationship orientated. They want to know how it will affect people, what people will have to do and whether people will belong. If they can see that people will benefit from the change they will be committed.

Directive people

This person needs to know exactly what is going to happen, what the rules will be and how the situation will change from the old to the new. Once they know precisely what will happen they will get involved quite forcefully.

(Rowe & Mason, 1987)

So how will you know who fits into each category? You could try asking them, although it's unlikely anyone will be able to fit themselves absolutely into one category. What you must assume is that you have someone with each personality type in your team. You will need to communicate frequently and also provide a broad amount of information to ensure that everyone gets the details they need to decide how they are going to respond.

Make sure that you plan the change carefully, identify someone to be responsible for every action and give them timescales to complete it. This will enable you to provide accurate information to your team. A sense of vagueness can make people assume the worst. People do not automatically think positively and will need some encouragement to do so.

You need to be able to identify exactly what will change and what will be different for them as individuals. As a line manager you may not be fully aware of the impact on every member of your team so talk to them and find out how things will be different for them. Once you have done that you will be able to determine who is going to lose what and help them to let go.

Bridges (Bridges & Bridges, 2000) provides a useful framework for managing through the neutral zone and he calls this 'The 4 Ps':

The 4 Ps

Purpose

Keep emphasising why the change is necessary. Be clear about your goals and the outcomes that will occur as a result of the change.

Picture

Describe what things will look like when the change is implemented and you have achieved your goals. If it is a physical change then get pictures or diagrams. If it is a new form, get examples.

Plan

Keep communicating your plan and updating everyone on the progress that is being made against the plan.

Part

Give everyone a part to play. If possible, involve people in the change or describe to them how they can help the change to be achieved. Make sure that they are clear what their role will be once the change is implemented.

Throughout this stage people will hark back to the past and issues will arise related to the past. Handle these rather than ignoring them as this can lead to dissatisfaction and unrest. Team working at this stage is really important as you want to avoid blame and encourage creativity.

As people move into the 'new beginnings' stage they will need preparation for new ways of working. Make sure that you behave in the new way. Role modelling is very important to ensure the sustainability of the change. Identify what training they will need to take on the new roles.

It is important to remember that it is normal to react to change in an emotional way. People will adapt to change at different rates. They will not move from one stage of transition to another together. Some will get frustrated with the rate of change because it is too slow, others because it is too fast. Encourage the team to work together and support each other.

The stages of change

The stages of change

The previous section discussed how people deal with change. This one looks at how change should be implemented. They are not separate processes but should happen in conjunction with one another.

There are a number of systems for implementing change these include Six Sigma and Lean (NHSIII, 2005), Total Quality Management and Re-engineering (Iles & Sutherland, 2001).

Whilst the models are different the stages of change are, however, similar.

Getting support

The first stage of implementing change is to find people to work with you. Consider the different personality types outlined above and identify the people in your team that will be the most appropriate to help you. You will not be able to introduce the change on your own, no matter how small.

Involve the key stakeholders as early as possible. Consider who has expertise in the field, who will be affected by the change and who will be involved in the change. If the implementation is likely to have resource implications or will impact more widely than your own team you will need to get the support of someone who has influence at a strategic level or has control of the budget. If the change is likely to have implications for other areas in your organisation involve someone who can help you to promulgate your work. If you are embarking on a change which will affect people outside your team you will need to involve them too. If it is likely to have an impact on patients then you should think about patient involvement (see Chapter 9).

Example: You are considering changing the way the team carries out the nursing handover. You will want to involve qualified nurses and unqualified nurses. You could also involve a student nurse, a housekeeper and perhaps the ward administrator. Involve patients to find out what they want and perhaps include your manager or matron who will help you share your work with other wards and departments.

Proving that you need to change

Why you need to change

Next you will need to identify why you need to change and what the current situation is. There are a number of different methods for this: observation of current practice, audit, a review of patients' notes, patient and staff interviews, data collection and process mapping.

Observation of care (RCN, 2005b)

This can be surprisingly helpful as people tend not to change their habits whilst being observed if the observation is carried out in the right way. It is a really useful tool for identifying areas that need improving.

Clinical audit

Clinical audit is defined as:

> a quality improvement process that seeks to improve patient care and outcomes through systematic review of care against explicit criteria and the implementation of change.

(CGST, 2005)

An audit of practice can be a really good way of finding out what needs to improve. For example, an audit of patient falls, observations or hand washing can reveal problems in the way care is delivered and can help you identify what needs to change. If you are considering undertaking an audit you should consult your organisation's clinical audit team who will be able to advise and help you.

Reviewing patients' notes

Going through past patients' notes and seeing what happened can help you identify issues with the patient pathway. It can be laborious but just reviewing a few sets of notes can give you a picture of what you want to know, depending on the kind of change you want to make.

Patient and staff interviews

This can be a useful tool if you want to get patient or staff perspectives. (See Chapter 9 for details about how to carry out patient interviews.) You may need to seek ethical approval to interview both staff and patients if the work is deemed to be research rather than audit. In order to be clear about your organisation's requirements, consult your clinical governance team or the lead for patient and public involvement. If the work is regarded as research, this can make the process more complex and it may not be necessary, so seek advice.

Consider who should carry out staff interviews. A line manager may not be appropriate as you might not get the most honest answers. You could ask a colleague from another area, a practice development nurse, someone from human resources or use an external facilitator.

Data collection

Providing facts and figures that support the need to change can be very powerful. You may not need to collect the data yourself; other departments in your organisation may already have it. For example, the directorate or division may have data about number of admissions and length of stay and the human resources department will have information about staff, such as turnover rates and sickness levels. The clinical governance team will be able to give you information in relation to incident reporting and audit results and the Patient Advice and Liaison Service (PALS) will be able to provide you with details of their concerns.

Process mapping

Process mapping (Modernisation Agency, 2005a) is simply getting people together to map the patients' journey. Everyone involved in the patient journey should be brought together including the patient themselves to carry out the exercise. The benefits of process mapping are that the discussion that takes place during the mapping brings people together and helps everyone to see what really happens, rather than what they assume happens. There may be people within your organisation who have the skills to facilitate process mapping who can help you set the exercise up.

Example: You want to identify what is currently happening during the nursing handover. The most suitable methods of finding out the current situation are observation and patient and staff interviews. Observations will tell you how long the handover takes, what is included or not included in the handover, who contributes and who doesn't, whether there are any learning opportunities and how confidential the process is.

Talking to staff will help you find out how useful they find the handover – whether they feel they are able to ask questions or challenge. Patients will be able to tell you if they feel involved, if the nurses looking after them know enough about them and so on.

Once you have an idea of what is currently happening you can start to think about what needs to change. You can get people involved because you can start to convince them about the need to change.

Visioning

Visioning

The next stage of the change management process is visioning. Generally, people find this quite difficult as it means thinking into the future, imagining what you would like to achieve in an ideal world. The importance of a vision is that it sets the direction for the team. Once you have decided what it is you want to achieve you can start to plan the steps you need to take to get there. It may take a number of years to achieve your vision, but it will help you to make the right decisions.

A vision or philosophy will not work if it is written down and stuck in a file or on a noticeboard where nobody looks at it. It needs to be a working tool that everyone is familiar with (Wells, 2005). It should be in line with the organisation's vision or mission statement and when drawing it up you should involve as many of the team as possible and it should be patient-focused.

Ask questions like:

'If this was the ideal ward to work in what would it look like?'
'If you could design this ward from scratch what would it look like?'
'If patients were designing the perfect ward, what would happen there?'

Example: You may develop a vision for the ward that encompasses broad principles, for example that all care will be patient-centred. This will emphasise the need to have a handover system that involves the patient and ensure that whatever system you put in place is in line with your vision.

Finding new ways of working

**Finding
new ways of
working**

Having established the current situation and what the ideal situation is you can then begin to think about how you are going to achieve it. You should establish what the evidence base is for the practice you want to change. This can be done by carrying out a literature search. Your trust librarian may do this for you or you could ask someone in your team who is undertaking an academic qualification to do this as part of their study. If it is clinical practice that you want to change then you should check national and local standards such as National Service Frameworks (www.dh.gov.uk) and NICE Guidelines, professional guidelines and trust policies and procedures. If there is evidence supporting a change in practice this will help to convince people to change.

Involve members of the team in the generation of ideas and to help you consider the impact on different members of the team.

Example: A literature search will tell you what methods other people have used for effective communication between staff on different shifts (giving handover), how they have implemented it, whether it worked or didn't work and why. Your trust policies will include a policy on confidentiality and documentation and the Nursing and Midwifery Council (NMC) has guidelines on record keeping and confidentiality. Members of your team may have worked in areas where they have experienced different methods of handover. Use their ideas and experience.

Testing out the idea

**Testing out
the idea**

Once you have agreed a possible solution you should pilot it. It is important that the pilot is just that, a pilot – a short-term test for a limited period that you then evaluate. You can use the PDSA cycle to help you do this (see Chapter 4).

It is important to communicate what the pilot entails and the results of the final evaluation to the whole team. It should demonstrate what has worked and what hasn't so that the planned change can be amended accordingly.

Example: Test out a method of handover on a small group of patients for one shift handover. If it wasn't successful find out why, amend the way it was done and test it again with the same number of patients on a different shift handover.

If it was successful, try it out on a larger number of patients or different shift patterns. Continue in this manner until you have achieved full implementation.

Finding resources

Finding resources

Most changes (but not all) will require some resources or a movement of resources from one area to another in the short term. Some will result in a saving in the long term either directly or indirectly.

If you need additional funding, either to pump prime the change or provide longer-term funding, you will need to write a business case. Each organisation will have a system for business planning with associated timescales. There may also be a template available for writing a business case. You should get help to develop your case and involve your manager and someone from the finance team. Find out who will be responsible for approving (or rejecting) it so that you can write the business case for your audience. Involve those who will have some influence at the beginning, before you start writing.

The business case should contain a summary stating what you are proposing. Keep it short and simple. Then set out the context – the background to the proposal and why you want to do it. How big will the change be and who is it going to affect? You will need to identify the costs of the proposal including staffing, training, equipment and stationery. It is important to highlight any savings that will be made and to do this you will need to know how much is currently being spent and what you think you will spend when the change has been made. Use examples from other organisations.

Finally, you need to identify the impact of the proposed change – what the benefits will be and how it will benefit patient care. What will be the impact on the organisation's share of the market and how will it affect patients' choice? Make sure the benefits are linked to the organisation's targets.

Emphasise the risks involved if the proposal is not supported. Your business case will provide a record of what you asked for and a record of the decisions made.

Once you have written the business case get someone else to read it to check that you have kept it simple and jargon free.

Implementation

Implementing change

Implementation is probably the hardest part of the change process as it rarely follows a smooth path; there are inevitably unforeseen events which will occur and detract from successful implementation.

Jick (1991) identifies a number of problems that companies experience when implementing change, such as overrunning the schedule, being distracted by competing crises, inadequate training and inadequate support. Consider the impact of the change on structure, technology and tasks as well as the people involved, as all these elements interact with each other and can impact on the success of the implementation (Leavitt (cited in Cork, 2005).

Example: You want to implement a new system of handover (which comes under Leavitt's definition of 'structure'). As well as thinking about the impact on staff and patients, you will need to consider the technology you might require, such as tape recorders for taped handovers or computers for electronic handover. Then you need to think about the task and how it will impact on other jobs. Will it encroach on mealtimes or interfere with drug rounds?

If you consider the impact on all aspects, you will minimise disruption and it will help you to plan the implementation realistically.

Ensuring sustainability

Sustaining change

We are all familiar with the scenario of implementing a change in practice and then members of the team reverting back to the old practice when we are off duty. That's what makes implementation so difficult.

Table 6.1 provides a checklist to help you get it right.

Improving patient outcomes

Table 6.1   **Change checklist**

Look at the current situation first	☐
Lead by example	☐
Provide strong leadership	☐
Provide training	☐
Develop a shared vision	☐
Create a sense of urgency	☐
Set goals and targets	☐
Find out the impact on people	☐
Set timescales	☐
Give maximum amount of warning for the change	☐
Explain the reasons for change	☐
Describe what will be different	☐
Keep patient-focused	☐
Involve people from the beginning	☐
Communicate	☐
Pilot and evaluate	☐
Ensure that there are short term successes	☐
Check how people are coping	☐

Example: You have decided to implement a walk round handover. You know that some people are not happy with the idea. Make sure that you have shared the results of the pilot with everyone. Always do a walk round handover yourself, keep reminding the team what the benefits are and keep it patient-focused. Keep monitoring the new system and involve the team in this. Keep checking how people feel about the change and support them. If you still don't have their commitment, find out what their objections are. Provide them with the evidence that led to this method being chosen.

Teams and strong leadership make change happen. Be honest with your team. Acknowledge that change is disruptive, give reassurance and recognise that people will respond emotionally.

Chapter 7
Implementing systems to support effective team working

Nursing plays a central role in patient safety and the quality of patient care and, as such, needs to be well organised in order to ensure that standards of care are high and errors are minimised. Ward leaders are in a powerful position to decide how the ward will be organised and therefore have a responsibility to ensure that there are systems and processes in place to enable the delivery of effective patient care.

A system can be defined as an organised, co-ordinated method. An Organisation with a Memory describes a system as:

> *a set of interdependent elements interacting to achieve a common aim. These elements may be both human and non-human.*
>
> (DH, 2000)

There are numerous systems and processes involved in running a ward, some of which have been discussed in other chapters (see Chapters 3, 4 and 5).

Others are discussed here. Systems and processes do not happen in a vacuum. They are all interlinked and small faults can accumulate and lead to accidents and incidents. Having no systems and processes in place can lead to confusion and error so it is important that everyone in the team is aware of how things are done.

Rostering

Rostering

Managing the 'off duty' can be one of the most stressful and time-consuming tasks that a ward leader has to do. It is also one of the most important systems to get right as having the right number of staff and skill mix at the right times is fundamental to the smooth and safe running of the ward or department. Anecdotally, many ward leaders do the off duty at home as this is the only place they can be guaranteed the time to do it. This is not ideal in itself but then when you return to work and put the neat, completed rota out for the staff you can be absolutely certain someone will want to change it! Here, then, are some suggestions to make 'doing the off duty' less of a struggle.

There are a number of different methods of rostering including self rostering, computerised rostering and rotational rostering (a roster which repeats every few weeks, for example a 12-week roster). However, some principles apply whatever method of rostering you are doing.

The rota should be available to staff at least four weeks in advance. It is unacceptable practice for nurses not to know what they are working until the last minute, as this can lead to at best dissatisfaction and at worst absenteeism and high staff turnover. Where possible, allow staff to swap shifts to give some last minute flexibility. Review the method of rostering and the shift patterns at least once a year. Identify the basic cover required for all shifts and make sure that this requirement is met. The rota is a legal document as it shows who was working when and so make sure it is legible and that a copy is kept on file.

The rota and shift patterns should reflect the European Working Time Directive which will be incorporated into hospital policies.

Self rostering

Much of the evidence about rostering shows that self rostering increases morale and performance and this has been recognised by the Department of Health (DH) who have produced *Working Lives: Programmes for Change: Team-based Self-rostering* (available at www.dh.gov.uk). Self rostering is a bottom-up approach to organising shift working and therefore gives nurses more ownership of the whole process. It is not necessarily a time saving exercise in the short term, but as staff become more familiar with it, it does become less onerous.

The benefits of self rostering are that staff have more control over what hours they are working, which means they are happier and more motivated. It has the potential to reduce turnover and sickness and, in the long run, frees up time for the ward leader. The team also need to work more closely together and help each other out, which should improve team working.

The ward leader needs to set parameters with the rest of the team. These will include:

- maximum and minimum staffing levels throughout the day and night and on particular days (fewer staff might be required when the workload is less)
- the grades and skill mix required at different times of the day and night
- how shortfalls will be addressed (usually this is the team's responsibility)
- the number of early and late shifts individuals are expected to work per week or month
- the number of weekends that staff are expected to work per month
- the requirements for working night shifts.

Dealing with requests is an issue whatever method of rostering you use. Team members should be given a limit to the number of requests they can make. My personal experience is that if you allow people to swap (within the same grade/competence), the number of requests is reduced. Requests at bank holidays (particularly Christmas and New Year) should also be restricted if allowed at all.

Setting separate restrictions for annual leave and study leave is also useful. You will need to consider:

- how much notice people need to give
- how many people can have annual leave at one time (within the skill mix)
- how many people can have study leave at the same time as annual leave is being taken.

These guidelines should be discussed and the rationale explained. They should then be agreed with the team.

Implementing self rostering

Start by involving all the staff. Decide on the parameters for your ward. Consider the impact on the delivery of patient care. Will it affect the way the care delivery is organised and, if so, how will you overcome this?

Agree with your team the method for completing the rota. How will you sort out discrepancies between the number of staff required to work a shift and the number who have selected the shift?

Get advice from your human resources department to ensure that you are being fair and reasonable.

Put annual leave, study leave and long-term sickness on the rota first, then put the rota out at least four weeks in advance for people to complete. The ward leader or a nominated other should act as arbitrator to prevent 'selfish' requests.

Implement self rostering on a trial basis so that you can adapt it if necessary and allow team members to give their feedback about the process. Set timescales for the trial and evaluate throughout.

The organisation of care delivery

Organising care delivery

Much has been written about models of nursing (Wimpenny, 2002; Aggleton & Chalmers, 2000; Tierney, 1998). This section will not focus on models but on the methods for delivering patient care. The method of care delivery is important for three reasons: the effectiveness of care, the quality of care and staff satisfaction. The main methods are functional nursing, team nursing or primary nursing.

Functional nursing or task nursing has been used for many years and was particularly popular when student nurses were part of the workforce. Tasks are divided and delegated according to people's abilities. One nurse is responsible for the observations, another for urinalysis and so on. The benefits of task allocation are that you can allocate a large number of tasks which can be accomplished in a relatively short space of time. It is also useful for training more junior staff. The disadvantages are that care becomes fragmented as no one person is aware of every aspect of a patient's care.

Team nursing has also been used for a number of years. The ward team is broken down into smaller teams, each led by a registered nurse. Each team is responsible for a group of patients or a geographical area. Patients may be allocated to a team for the duration of their stay or the team may change.

The advantages to team nursing are that, as a ward leader, you can use each member according to their strengths. It encourages team working and enables decisions to be made nearer to the patient.

There is some evidence to suggest that staff satisfaction is increased with team nursing (Gullick, 2004). The problems with team nursing are that you need skilled team leaders, an adequate number of staff and the right skill mix for it to work.

With **primary nursing** a named registered nurse is accountable for a patient throughout their stay in hospital. In this method of organisation the focus is on the patient giving the nurse an opportunity to form a relationship with the patient and their family. As one nurse has responsibility for all the care of the patient they have greater autonomy. There is some evidence that where primary nursing is implemented nurse retention is increased although this has been challenged (Kangas *et al.*, 1999; Steven, 1999).The disadvantages to primary nursing are that you need to have experienced staff to take on the role of primary nurse and you also need a good skill mix.

For each method you may decide to use, there are some things you should consider.

Functional nursing

As ward leader you will need to take responsibility for the delegated tasks. You will need to think how you will motivate team members and create a feeling of autonomy and responsibility which does not come automatically with this method of nursing. Communication is really important to avoid the sense of fragmentation. Where possible, you will need to rotate the tasks to create variety and promote learning.

Team nursing

The ward leader's role in team nursing is to act as a consultant to the team leaders. Responsibility for decision making should be delegated to the team leaders who will organise their team. The team leader needs to know how to delegate appropriately. Consider the size of the team and number of patients each team will be responsible for. Will the composition of the teams change or will there be continuity? How will you allocate the workload amongst the teams?

Primary nursing

You need to have staff who are willing to participate so you need to work with your team to get them on board. You will need to provide support and education to all members of the multi-disciplinary team to ensure that it works.

Primary nurses need to be experienced and willing to take on the responsibility of the role.

Handover

Handover

Handover is defined by the British Medical Association (BMA) as:

the transfer of professional responsibility and accountability for some or all aspects of care for a patient, or group of patients, to another person or professional group on a temporary or permanent basis.

(BMA, 2005)

Nursing handovers generally take place between each shift and when new staff come on duty. It is the primary method of communication during the shift. Handovers directly affect the delivery of care for the following shift (Thurgood, 1995; Pothier *et al.*, 2005) and yet they can be ritualistic, ineffective and time consuming. They can also be extremely nerve-wracking for junior staff and students.

There are four recognised methods of handover: written, tape recorded, bedside and verbal. Research by Pothier *et al. (op. cit.)* showed that when handover is purely verbal most of the information passed from one shift to another is lost and that if staff are allowed to take notes less information is lost. The most reliable method is using a pre-printed typed sheet. Using tape recorders can save time and is particularly useful if you have people coming on duty at different times.

Sexton showed that the lack of written guidelines as to what should be included in handover meant that the content was often vague and confusing (Sexton, 2004). It was felt that guidelines would also help reduce the time spent in handover. Much of the research shows that nurses do not always use the nursing notes to give handover, more usually referring to their own notes. This means that giving handover and updating nursing records are seen as two separate activities. This also results in not all the relevant information being passed on. Davies *et al.* piloted a template for handover which also doubled as a care sheet and was then kept in the patient notes (Davies *et al.*, 2006). Giving handover at the bedside means that the discussion is focused on the patient and the patient can be encouraged to take part. Confidentiality need not be an issue if the diagnosis is not discussed in front of other patients.

More recently some hospitals are developing electronic nurse handover and this includes systems for handover. Some of the benefits of electronic systems that are linked to the hospital network is that you can standardise the format of the handover, reduce staff time involved in handover and link to other parts of the patient documentation to get information (DH, forthcoming).

A good handover will increase patient safety, continuity of care and avoid repetition for patients. It should also be an opportunity for education for both staff and patients. Whatever method of handover is used the following principles should be adhered to:

- involve the patient
- maintain confidentiality by discussing nursing care only at the bedside
- destroy any written lists at the end of each shift (before leaving the ward)
- do not use bed numbers or bays to identify patients
- avoid jargon and abbreviations
- the incoming shift should not be passive recipients of information but should challenge and ask questions
- students giving handover must be accompanied by their mentor or senior nurse from the shift
- avoid interruptions
- do not be subjective, but factual and accurate
- encourage learning
- use nursing notes.

Effective meetings

Effective meetings

The commonest complaint that I hear from ward leaders about their meetings is that nobody attends or that it is the same people attending each time. In theory, people will attend a meeting if they find it useful, but this is oversimplifying things when you are dealing with a team who work shifts and when you have to provide cover for the ward while the meeting is taking place. However, there are some things you can do to make your meetings more effective. Meetings will be more successful if they are well chaired, the agenda is well prepared and genuine progress is made on agenda items from one meeting to the next.

Firstly, consider the purpose of the meeting and if it is unnecessary, don't meet! If the information can be circulated to the relevant people by email, letter or a notice then do it that way. Preferably use more than one method.

Communication is vitally important to the morale and performance of the team so if you are going to meet make sure that you are clear about the objectives for the meeting. Set some terms of reference (see Appendix 4), agree these with the team and ensure that they are circulated to everyone. At induction, make sure that each new team member is given details of the meetings and their role.

Develop some ground rules such as:

- confidentiality
- punctuality
- participation
- sharing information from the meeting
- actions being completed.

Having agreed the purpose of the meeting, decide who will participate and be careful whom you exclude as this can be divisive. A team meeting should be for all members of the team. A meeting for another purpose may not need to include everyone. Try not to cancel meetings as this will send out the message that they are not important.

Setting the agenda

An agenda is important because it provides a framework for the meeting. It should be distributed in advance of the meeting to allow participants to prepare. You can use it as a checklist in advance to ensure that you have prepared correctly and during the meeting it can be used to ensure you have covered everything. Ask people what they want on the agenda. A useful way to do this is to put the agenda on a noticeboard where staff can access it. Make sure they put their name against the item and that they will be present at the meeting to discuss it. If people put unsuitable items on the agenda – subjects that are relevant only to the minority – then arrange to discuss this with them outside the meeting.

Preparing for the meeting

Set dates well in advance and, barring a clinical emergency, make sure that the meeting goes ahead on time. Choose a venue where there will be fewest interruptions. Arrange the room in a semicircle or circle and, if possible, provide refreshments even if only glasses of water.

You could display the agenda on a flipchart or white board, particularly if people may have forgotten to bring their copies. Have spare copies of the agenda and notes from the previous meeting.

Conducting the meeting

The ward leader does not have to chair the meeting, but it is quite a skill to chair a meeting effectively, so use someone who is confident and support them prior to and at the meeting. Make sure that you provide them with feedback at the end. The role of the chairperson is to keep the meeting on track and make sure the meeting achieves its purpose. The chair must be impartial and assertive.

If an issue comes up that dominates the meeting inappropriately then suggest either another meeting or postpone it to the following agenda. If a decision is required and the group are being indecisive, the chairperson should push for a decision, if necessary taking a vote. If someone is contributing too much, try and encourage others to participate. Say things like 'Mary, you've had a lot of experience with this,. What do you think?' or 'Thanks for that Rob. Could we just see what everyone else thinks?' Going round the room and asking each person their thoughts is a useful method but can be intimidating for some.

Identify actions for people and give them timescales. If the meeting is going over time ask the group which items can be left until the next meeting. At the end of each item summarise the key points and any decisions made and make sure the meeting starts and finishes on time.

Minutes or action notes

You must record what has happened in the meeting. The note taker will find it difficult to take notes and to contribute. Ideally, ask someone who is not part of the team to take on this task (you could swap this role with another ward) or rotate the job between members of the team.

Minutes are a more detailed record of what took place at the meeting. Action notes simply identify what needs to be done, when and who by. There are templates for both in Appendix 4.

Give feedback to all attendees. Take time to evaluate the meeting at the end. You can do that simply by going round the room and asking each person what went well about the meeting and what didn't.

Following the meeting

Make sure the meeting notes are copied up and circulated or available to all members of the team. Any items which need a follow up or were not discussed should be added to the agenda for the following meeting. Follow up any delegated actions and make sure that people know what is expected of them. Make sure actions are carried out; a meeting which doesn't lead to any action will be very unpopular!

You won't improve attendance at the meetings immediately but with persistence the attitude to meetings amongst the team will change and they will not want to miss out.

Managing sickness

Managing sickness

On average, employee sickness and absence costs employers £601 per employee per year or nine days for every member of staff per year (CIPD, 2005b). Sickness and absence also puts additional strain on the remaining team and can result in the use of temporary staff.

Successful strategies to reduce sickness rely heavily on the manager's belief that the problem can be, at least partly, solved. The most common approaches to managing sickness include return to work interviews, setting trigger points and keeping records. The disciplinary procedure (see Chapter 5) can also be instigated for individuals who persistently take time off (Johnson *et al.*, 2003).

Your trust will have policies and procedures for time off work including sickness. You should refer to these and to your human resources team to ensure that you manage individuals within the policies and the law. The two acts which cover the management of sickness and absence are the Employment Act 2002 and the Employment Act 2002 (Dispute Resolution) Regulations 2004 but there are other laws which you need to comply with including the Data Protection Act and the Disability Act.

To help reduce sickness and absence in your team there are some systems you should have in place.

Measurements

As discussed in Chapter 9, measurements can help identify a problem and provide a focus for the team to tackle. ACAS (2005) provide the following formula for calculating the amount of sickness in your team:

$$\frac{\text{Total absence (hours or days) in the period}}{\text{Possible total (hours or days) in the period}} \times 100$$

If the total hours lost in a week is 22 and the possible total hours in that week were 888 (24 members of staff working 37 hours each) then the formula is:

$$\frac{22}{888} \times 100 = 2.5\%$$

This formula is useful to demonstrate the amount of sickness within the team and can be used to benchmark against other teams.

The Bradford factor

The Bradford factor is an absence measurement tool, thought originally to have been employed by the Incomes Data Services in the 1980s.

Short-term sickness can be very disruptive as it doesn't allow the planning that long-term sickness does. If it isn't dealt with then it can give out the message that taking the odd day off is acceptable. There is also no requirement to have short-term sickness (less than seven days) certified and this can lead to suspicion about the cause of the absence.

The Bradford factor measures an employee's irregularity of attendance. The formula is:

S x S x D = Bradford score

S is the number of spells of absence in the last year and D is the number of days of absence during the last year. For an employee who has 12 days absence in one year, on a different number of occasions, the calculations are as follows:

1 absence of 12 days = 1 x 1 x 12 = 12 points

2 absences of 6 days = 2 x 2 x 6 = 24 points

6 absences of 2 days = 6 x 6 x 2 = 72 points

The person having the most number of absences, rather than the longer time off sick, receives the most points.

You need to set triggers in order to make use of this tool. For example, you need to set how many points an individual will need to score before you interview them and how many points they will they need to trigger an occupational health referral or disciplinary action. Your trust may already have guidance for this. If not you should get advice from your human resources department.

The Bradford factor should not be used in isolation, but in conjunction with the other methods outlined here and in conjunction with your trust policies and human resources department.

Return to work interviews

Every time an employee returns to work following a period of sickness, no matter how short, they should be interviewed by the line manager. The employee must be told the reason for the meeting and it must be carried out in confidence. It should start by ascertaining the well being of the employee. The absence should be brought to the attention of the individual and they should be given opportunity to discuss their problems and any support that they need. The meeting should be recorded in the personal file. A return to work interview form is available in Appendix 5.

Long-term sickness

The main principle of managing long-term sickness is that you must keep in touch with the individual. This serves two purposes: it allows you to provide support for the individual and to keep up-to-date with progress regarding their return to work. You will need to involve your human resources team and occupational health. Your trust policies will guide you through the management of people who are off sick for long periods, providing opportunities for the individual to be assessed before they return to work.

To manage sickness and absence successfully every member of the team should be aware of the procedure. Monitor sickness and share statistics (but not the Bradford factor score) with the team. Be consistent and caring but use the disciplinary process if needed. Ensure that the whole team knows that you are proactively managing sickness and that you are treating everyone the same. Sending out a firm message will help to keep sickness to a minimum.

Complaints and compliments

Complaints & compliments

Complaints analysis

Complaints about healthcare from patients and their relatives are now a reality. The number of complaints received by NHS hospitals and community services in 2004–5 was 90,413 and staff attitude is the biggest cause of complaint after clinical treatment (Health and Social Care Information Centre press release, 30.11.05, available at www.ic.nhs.uk/news). The NHS has a standard complaints procedure which has to be adhered to by all trusts.

Every ward leader must be aware of the complaints that are received about their service. It is easy to take complaints personally but it is important to learn from what they say. Most trusts will provide an analysis of the complaints received with a breakdown by area and topic but if this does not happen it is important to undertake your own complaints analysis. This will help you identify areas for improvement and enable you to celebrate success and provide positive feedback to team members. It will also help you to become more proactive and less reactive.

Start by counting the number of complaints you receive and compare this with the number of patients you treat. You can then make comparisons with other wards and with previous months or years. Whilst complaints are rarely about one topic, it is possible to categorise them. The Health and Social Care Information Centre (HSCIC) uses a number of topics to analyse complaints, but you could equally use the benchmark headings from *Essence of Care* (DH, 2001b) or a combination of the two. Both are listed below. (See Appendix 6 for a complaints analysis pro forma.)

HSCIC topics for complaints analysis

HSCIC topics for complaints analysis

- Admissions, discharge and transfer arrangements
- Aids and appliances, equipment, premises (including access)
- Appointments, delay/cancellation (out-patient)
- Appointments, delay/cancellation (in-patient)
- Attitude of staff
- All aspects of clinical treatment
- Communication/information to patients (written and oral)
- Consent to treatment
- Complaints handling
- Patients' privacy and dignity
- Patients' property and expenses
- Personal records (including medical and/or complaints)
- Failure to follow agreed procedures
- Patients' status, discrimination (for example, racial, gender or age)
- Transport (ambulances and other)
- Hotel services (including food)

Amended by the author from www.ic.nhs.uk/news

Essence of care benchmarks

Essence of Care benchmarks

- Continence and bladder and bowel care
- Personal and oral hygiene
- Food and nutrition
- Pressure ulcers
- Privacy and dignity
- Record keeping
- Safety of clients with mental health needs in acute mental health and general hospital settings
- Principles of self-care
- Promoting health

You can also categorise complaints by seriousness. Your trust will probably have a system for doing this so check their policy. Complaints can be graded as minor, moderate or serious (Table 7.1).

Table 7.1   **Grading complaints**

Minor	Moderate	Serious
minimal or no discomfort	semi-permanent harm	major permanent harm
non-permanent harm	potential for some discomfort	major clinical intervention
no increased length of stay	slight increase in the length of stay	unscheduled return to theatre
only minor clinical intervention required	admission to hospital	unscheduled admission to ITU/CCU
	moderate clinical intervention	the potential for severe discomfort
	immediate surgery	

Moderate and serious complaints must be reported to someone more senior according to your hospital policy.

You should not only analyse written complaints but consider verbal complaints and Patient Advice and Liaison Service (PALS) concerns too. Analysing complaints will help you to benchmark yourself against other wards and organisations. It will also help you to identify where to focus your energy on improving the service. Make sure that you identify changes that you have made as a result of complaints and feed these back to both complainants and staff.

Compliments

Don't forget to analyse the compliments you receive too. Your ward will receive cards and verbal compliments. Record and analyse these and feedback the results to your staff. This might be done in a simple chart on the wall or a notice on a noticeboard.

Number of compliments/complaints			
	May	June	July
☺	27	15	18
☹	2	1	1

Improving patient outcomes

Incident reporting

Chapter 4 discusses the need for a change in culture in the NHS in order to reduce the number of patients harmed unintentionally whilst in its care (estimated at 10%). The National Patient Safety Agency (NPSA) reports that 85,342 patient safety incidents were reported up until March 2005. Of these, 68% resulted in no harm to the patient but about 100 led to severe harm or death (NPSA, 2005). On average, 22% adverse incidents go unreported (Beckford-Ball, 2005).

In Seven Steps to Patient Safety the NPSA (2004) outlines the need for incident reporting and root cause analysis in order to create a learning culture and the reduction of harm to patients. Every registered nurse has a responsibility and statutory duty to report adverse incidents particularly where patients are at risk (NMC, 2004). A patient safety incident is defined as:

> *any unintended or unexpected incident which could have or did lead to harm for one or more patients receiving NHS funded healthcare.*

(NPSA, 2004).

There are a number of things which stop staff reporting incidents, these include:

- fear of blame
- a sense of failure
- scepticism about the benefits of reporting incidents
- fear of reprisal
- lack of trust
- lack of time.

(Bird, 2005)

Each trust will have an incident reporting system with which you should make sure that you are familiar. This will include incident reporting forms and a policy. The focus of incident reporting should be on problem solving and not blame. Staff should understand the purpose of incident reporting and should receive information about what has happened to the report and what actions will be taken to prevent a repeat of the incident. Your organisation will probably analyse incidents and carry out investigations if necessary but you may want to have systems in place to analyse reports on a local basis. The benefits of this are that you will identify problems early, you will be able to give feedback to your team quickly and you will be able to rectify the problem or raise awareness in the right places.

Your reporting system may mean that you keep a copy of incident reports on the ward. You could set up a simple database using your computer or even a table that you complete by hand. The important thing about incident reporting is identifying the underlying cause. There are four different categories of causation:

- working environment (including equipment, light, space)
- individual (knowledge, skills, behaviour and health)
- organisational (including financial constraints, policies, protocols, communication and culture)
- external (including statutory requirements and professional bodies).

To determine the cause of an incident you need to determine the sequence of events that led to the incident. You need to identify the conditions which created the incident (causal factors) and understand the interaction between the sequence of events and the causal factors. For example:

A staff nurse administers the wrong drug to a patient.

Sequence of events
1. The staff nurse is undertaking a drug round on the night shift.
2. The phone rings during the drug round (just as she gets to the patient who has received the incorrect medication).
3. The patient asks if he can go to the toilet.
4. The nurse picks up the wrong bottle and gives the patient the medication.
5. When she puts the bottle back in the trolley she realises her mistake.

Causal factors
- The staff nurse has worked overtime this week and is tired.
- The light in the bay is not working.
- There are two similar looking bottles of tablets containing different types of medication kept together in the trolley.

Interaction between events and causal factors

The staff nurse was tired and the light was dim, she was distracted by the telephone and the patient. She said she felt stressed and was in a rush to finish the medicine round. She was familiar with the drug trolley and knew what the bottle looked like that contained the tablets she was looking for. She did not check the label on the bottle properly.

The patient was not aware that it was the wrong tablet and did not come to any harm. The nurse explained to the patient what had happened and gave her apologies.

In this scenario it would be easy to apportion blame to the staff nurse and even start a disciplinary procedure. But this would not only be excessively punitive to the nurse but would create a lack of trust amongst the rest of the team and deter them from reporting the error. And it would not solve the problem. If the patient was unaware of the mistake and no harm came to him the nurse could easily have decided not to report the incident (to avoid punishment). In that case the team would be none the wiser and future errors where more harm might result would not be prevented.

By undertaking a root cause analysis you can determine what led to the error and develop an action plan to prevent it from happening again.

Firstly, you should focus on solving the problem rather than on apportioning blame. A useful tool for identifying the underlying cause is to ask 'why' five times. This problem solving approach was made popular in the 1970s by the Toyota Production System and has been adopted widely by the NHS (NPSA, 2006).

Using the scenario above, this is how it would work:

Possible cause 1

Staff nurse tired on duty

Why?

1. She worked overtime on 3 shifts prior to this shift.
2. The ward was short staffed throughout the week. Unable to book agency or bank staff.
3. Ward short staffed due to annual leave.
4. Too many people had booked annual leave at once.
5. No rules in place to restrict number of people on annual leave.

Possible cause 2

Two bottles of tablets look the same

Why?

1. Labels on bottles are the same colour.
2. Tablets made by the same manufacturer.

Possible cause 3

Light not working in bay

Why?

1. Bulb not replaced.
2. Form completed to report bulb not working but bulb still not replaced.
3. Form not sent to estates department.
4. Ward clerk on holiday.
5. Isn't there another method of reporting the bulb?

Possible cause 4

Staff nurse rushing drug round

Why?

1. She was late starting the round and someone else is waiting for the trolley
2. The nurse had to wait for the drug trolley
3. Another nurse was using the trolley
4. There are four teams to do their drugs and only one trolley
5. Why is there only one trolley?

The result of asking 'why?' five times leads the investigator to a number of changes that could be made to help prevent a similar incident happening again.

- You could restrict the amount of overtime staff work.
- Rules need to be put in place to restrict the amount of people who are on annual leave at any one time.
- You could discuss with pharmacy the possibility of labelling the medications differently or putting them in different bottles.
- You could look into alternative ways to get light bulbs replaced or have a method of reporting when the ward clerk is not on duty.
- You could have two drug trolleys.
- You could find another way of organising drug administration, such as self-administration.

This exercise must be followed by action planning to ensure that the situation is resolved. If resources are needed to implement change, for example funding for an extra drug trolley without room in your budget to do so, you will need to raise this as part of the business planning process (see Chapter 6).

Chapter 8
Involving patients in their care

When patients come into contact with the NHS they can be at their most vulnerable and emotional. Many feel anxious and scared and describe how the situation can be made worse by the way they are treated by healthcare professionals. Patients describe what they want from the NHS in *Now I Feel Tall* (DH, 2005):

- good treatment in a comfortable, caring and safe environment, delivered in a calm and reassuring way
- information to make choices, to feel confident and to feel in control
- to be talked to and listened to as an equal
- to be treated with honesty, respect and dignity.

For a number of years patient involvement has been central to government policy in a bid to overcome negative feedback and meet patients' expectations. The following documents outline how this will be achieved:

Working for Patients (DH, 1989)

The Patient's Charter (DH, 1991)

The NHS Plan (DH, 2000)

Our National Health: A Plan for Action, a Plan for Change (Scottish Executive, 2000)

The Health and Social Care Act 2001 (DH, 2001a)

Creating a Patient-led NHS: Delivering the NHS Improvement Plan (DH, 2003)

Strengthening Accountability Involving Patients and the Public: Practice Guidance (Section 11 of the Health and Social Care Act 2001) (DH, 2003a)

A Stronger Local Voice: A Framework for Creating a Stronger Local Voice in the Development of Health and Social Care (DH, 2006a)

Our Health, Our Care, Our Say (DH, 2006b)

Improving patient outcomes

Section 11 of the Health and Social Care Act 2001 places a duty on NHS trusts to involve and consult patients in the planning, development and provision of services. Involving patients and public in health services is about changing the relationship between patients and professionals from a paternalistic approach to one where patients are empowered and can participate actively in their care. The benefits of patient involvement have been widely acknowledged (Coulter, 2002; DH, 2004b; RCN, 2004) and include increased patient satisfaction, reduced stress and fatigue and increased symptom control. Self care can also lead to reduced attendances, as in-patients and out-patients, and can therefore be cost-efficient. There are also benefits for health professionals as they develop a greater understanding of patients' problems and gain greater trust and credibility.

The biggest driver for involving patients is that it will lead to an improvement in the way services are delivered. Asking patients what they need and changing the way care is delivered will lead to a system that is patient-focused. The Department of Health (DH) has a number of public service agreements which are a clear statement of what the government is trying to achieve. Two are related to patient involvement. For 2003–6:

> to enhance accountability to patients and public and secure sustained national improvements in patient experience as measured by independently validated surveys.

and for 2005–8:

> to secure sustained national improvements in NHS patients' experience by 2008, as measured by independently validated surveys ensuring that individuals are fully involved in decisions about their healthcare, including choice of provider.

These have led to the NHS Patient Survey programme. The programme is delivered by the Picker Institute and managed by the Healthcare Commission on behalf of the Department of Health. A number of different surveys are carried out each year. The National Patient Survey is distributed to all acute and specialist trusts across England. In 2005, 169 acute trusts were involved. The response rate from patients was 59%. The survey has ten sections:

- Admission
- Hospital and ward
- Doctors

- Nurses
- Care and treatment
- Pain
- Operations and procedures
- Leaving hospital
- Overall (including how well doctors and nurses work together)
- About you and response rates.

The ten sections are based on five themes: access and waiting; safe, high quality co-ordinated care; better information, more choice; building closer relationships; and clean, comfortable environment (DH, 2005).

The results from each trust can be viewed on the Picker Institute website along with the programme for planned surveys (www.pickereurope.org).

As well as patient surveys the government has implemented a Patient Advice and Liaison Service (PALS) in every trust to help resolve patients' and carers' concerns as early as possible. 'Patient and public involvement' forums have also been established in every trust to obtain the views of local people. In 2002, the DH also put the Expert Patient Programme into place. This is based on research undertaken in the USA that showed if people with chronic diseases are allowed to manage their own condition there is a positive impact on the disease and their quality of life. The programme is supported by volunteer tutors and is delivered over six weeks. Participants attend for two and half hours a week and cover a number of topics including diet, medication and pain management. Details of the programme are available at www.expertpatients.nhs.uk.

The ability of trusts to deliver patient-focused care will also be monitored as part of the Annual Health Check (DH, 2004f).

Levels of involvement

Levels of involvement

Brearly describes patient involvement as:

being allowed to become involved in a decision-making process or in the delivery and evaluation of a service, or even simply being consulted on an issue of care such as activities of daily living, pain management or treatment options.

(Brearly, 1990)

There are different levels of patient involvement:

giving information – which may include written and verbal formats such as leaflets, reports, and education

consultation – which consists of a continuing dialogue in order to learn and respond to each other, for example discussions about service development, patient surveys and complaints

participation – involving patients directly in decision making, for example in care planning and evaluating care.

In wards and departments, patient involvement can operate at all three levels. For example, you will provide patients with leaflets about their condition, what to bring in to hospital and what will happen to them in hospital. Nurses will teach patients how to administer medication and what diet and exercise they should take.

You may consult patients about their stay in hospital by administering questionnaires or running focus groups. If you are considering making changes to the service you deliver, such as changing the visiting hours, you should first consult patients and their relatives to obtain their views.

Finally, you can involve patients in decision making by including them in ward rounds, allowing them to participate in care planning or managing their medication.

Before embarking on patient involvement it is important to check that what you are doing is not regarded as research or involves any ethical issues that you need to consider. You should therefore consult your organisation's clinical governance team or your lead for patient and public involvement who will be able to guide you through the research governance issues.

Blocks to involving patients

Blocks to involvement

Patient involvement or participation should be seen as a process that is part of care giving (Tutton, 2005). Unfortunately, it can sometimes be viewed as an additional task for healthcare professionals to do and therefore time-consuming. However, if viewed as part of the care-giving process, any additional time it takes should be minimal. Making improvements to the service as a result of patient feedback may also mean that you are able to save time by reducing the number of complaints you have to deal with.

Stereotyping patients or making assumptions about them can also limit the amount of patient involvement. Assuming that patients are too young or too old or do not have the capacity to make decisions can be a mistake. Using creative methods such as drawing and texting means that most patients can participate in their care to some degree or other. Where it is impossible to involve the patient themselves – such as in the case of babies or patients that are unconscious – relatives or carers must be involved to make sure you are still able to get to know the patient. *Now I Feel Tall* (DH, 2005) describes a number of case studies of the ways in which children's and people with learning difficulties' opinions have been successfully sought.

Some professionals find patient involvement a challenge to their power or status or that they don't feel they have the skills to develop closer relationships with patients. It is important that all staff members are supported in order to change their behaviour or attitude. Once staff take on the responsibility of being more patient-centred they will find their role more satisfying (Binnie & Titchen, 1999).

There are a number of ways you can encourage patient involvement on your ward.

Encouraging involvement

Patient-centred care

Patient-centred care

Patient-centred care is the sharing of the management of an illness between the patient and professionals (Bauman *et al.*, 2003). It is moving away from task-centred care to patient-focused care. Reed and McCormack cite four factors that older people have identified to enable patient-centred care (Reed & McCormack, 2005). They would like nurses to anticipate their needs, rather than remind them of their vulnerability and dependency, and to help them maintain their autonomy. Finally, patients would like nurses to be understanding and attentive rather than patronising. Binnie and Titchen (1999) also stress the importance of anticipating patients' needs and avoiding 'over hasty categorisation' or stereotyping (Binnie and Titchen, 1999). To be able to anticipate patient needs you and your team must understand what's important to them, their feelings and how they want to live their life (Tutton, 2005), and to discover this information you will need to employ some of the methods outlined later in this chapter.

To create a team which delivers patient-centred care you will need to build the right culture. Research undertaken into the theory-practice gap in relation to newly qualified nurses (Maben and Latter, 2006) shows that newly qualified nurses often feel discouraged from becoming involved with patients. Few of them experienced role modelling by senior nurses and, although they aspired to holistic nursing, they felt discouraged from getting too involved with patients. The increased workload of nurses along with increased expectations means that senior nurses have to prioritise and Maben and Latter feel this has led to prioritising the needs of the many over individual needs. Surveys of NHS patients in 2004 found that 47% of in-patients would have liked more input and choice in decisions about their care (Picker, 2005) so the ethos of ward nurses does need to be changed.

Role modelling is an important factor in developing the culture in a team (see Chapter 4) and will need to focus on the following factors:

- good communications with patients (listening and talking)
- understanding the needs of the patients
- keeping patients informed and involved in their care.
- explicit standards of care
- politeness and respect
- the ability to respond flexibly to individuals' needs
- responding to the needs of patients by ensuring services are improved.

The organisation of nursing is also important (see Chapter 7). Your method must support the continuity of care. Primary nursing is therefore the ideal way to enable the delivery of patient-centred care. An adapted team model could work if it is established in such a way that nurses are responsible for the same patients on each shift. Continuity of care allows nurses to develop relationships with patients and increases the amount of involvement patients and families have in their care.

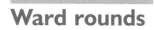

Ward rounds

Ward rounds

Traditionally, medical ward rounds are conducted by the consultant and his entourage. More recently the trend is toward multi-disciplinary rounds and the evidence is that where the whole team is involved length of stay is reduced (Moroney *et al.*, 2006). Often the ward round is the only opportunity the patient has to have a conversation with the consultant. The number of people participating in a ward round can be intimidating to the patient and so a conscious effort is required to ensure that they are able to participate. Moroney provides a useful checklist for the team to complete which helps ensure that everyone has had a chance to contribute to the discussion.

Ideally, numbers should be kept to a minimum. This will also help to secure the patient's privacy and dignity. Patients should also know in advance when the rounds will take place as this will enable them to prepare. Consider also allowing relatives and carers to be present during ward rounds, but check first what the patient wants.

Anecdotally, many nurses feel that participating in the medical round is not a nursing priority but this can lead to miscommunication and prevent the nurse from taking part in decision making and acting as a patient advocate. Participating in a multi-disciplinary ward round that includes the patient will help to ensure that not only are the right decisions made but that they are timely too.

Care planning

Care planning

Care planning is a fundamental way of involving patients in their care. It involves assessing a patient's needs, interpreting the information and then identifying their actual or potential problems. It is then important to identify what the patient's goals are. The whole process is about the interaction with patients and, if appropriate, their carers. Commonly the evaluation of care plans is carried out by the nurse on her own but this is an ideal time to discuss the care with the patient and to plan subsequent care.

To promote the involvement of patients in care planning keep care plans by the bedside and encourage nurses to update the documentation by the bed, with the patient. Try to be open and honest, avoid using medical jargon and use open-ended questions (see Chapter 5).

Integrated care pathways

Johnson defines an integrated care pathway as an amalgamation of:

all the anticipated elements of care and treatment of all members of the multi-disciplinary team, for a patient or client of a particular case-type or grouping within an agreed timeframe, for the achievement of agreed outcomes. Any deviation from the plan is documented as a 'variance'; the analysis of which provides information for the review of current practice.

(Johnson, 1997)

It is an evidence-based document used as a tool to set standards for a specific group of patients. It should form all of the documentation and is not an additional piece of paper for professionals to complete. It should be used by the whole multi-disciplinary team and should include a care plan and a timeframe and allow for variations.

The benefits of implementing a care pathway are numerous. It will support the implementation of clinical governance in a number of ways, including ensuring practice is evidence-based and patient-centred. It will help to improve morale and team building. The pathway can be used as a teaching aid for staff and patients and will also help to reduce the risk of clinical negligence.

Patients can be involved with care pathways in different ways. They must be involved in their development to ensure that they are patient-focused. They should be encouraged to complete parts of the document and it can be used to inform them about the care plan.

Examples of care pathways and a step-by-step approach to implementing them can be found at www.library.nhs.uk.

Self-medication

Self-medication

The traditional methods of drug administration can be problematic: drug trolleys become overloaded with medicines and specific medications can be difficult to find, there are numerous interruptions and the nurse may not be familiar with each patient's medical history (Reid *et al.*, 2002).

Self-administration of medication benefits both the patient and the nurse. It allows the patient to maintain their independence and can help improve the relationship between the nurse and the patient. In addition, the timings of administration can be more precise and the patient's knowledge and understanding of the medication increases. There is evidence to show that introducing self-medication can increase the efficiency of patient discharge, increase patient and staff satisfaction and lead to a reduction in medication errors (Grantham *et al.*, 2006).

There are three levels of self-medication:

1. medications are administered by the registered nurse
2. the administration of medications is directly supervised by the registered nurse
3. the administration of medications is indirectly supervised by the registered nurse.

Patient education should underpin all three levels. Patients are assessed according to predetermined criteria to determine which level they should be on. These will usually include that the patient is responsible for administering their own medication at home or in the community, that they are over 16 and that they fully understand the scheme. It will also include whether the patient is able to open the cabinet, read and open the containers and understand the purpose and the side effects of the medication.

Before implementing self-administration of medication in your area, check your trust's policies. You will need to work closely with the pharmacist and medical staff. You will need a secure place to keep the medications at the bedside as well as the supporting documentation (consent forms, protocols and information booklets). You will also need to ensure that there is education for nurses who will be working with the scheme.

Implementing a change in the administration of medications will require change management skills (see Chapter 6) as there may be some resistance from nurses. Nurses may have some concerns about the time involved in supporting patients to self-medicate (Deegan *et al.*, 2005). Generally the additional time is required at the beginning as everyone becomes familiar with the process. In the long term, the benefits make the additional time spent worthwhile.

Patient information

Patient information

A number of different formats can be used to give patients information, including video and audio tapes, posters and leaflets. All information should be easily accessible and clear. Consider patients whose first language is not English and those with visual or hearing impairments. *The Essence of Care* (DH, 2001a) provides useful guidelines for implementing patient information. Include patients and carers in the development of patient information to ensure that it meets their needs.

Leaflets are a useful way of providing patients with information and can be produced at a relatively low cost. Check whether your trust has a policy for written information for patients. It may also provide a template for the layout. The Plain English Campaign provides guidelines for developing patient information on its website (www.plainenglish.co.uk). The campaign advises that you use black or blue ink on a white background. Font size should be 12 point or 14 point if it is likely to be used by people with visual impairment. Paragraphs should be short and sentences kept to 20 words or less. You should use active rather than passive sentences, for example:

'You will have your blood pressure recorded every hour.'

becomes

'A nurse will record your blood pressure every hour.'

You should also make the information personal, for example:

'Sister Jones and her team welcome you to Felix Ward.'

as opposed to

'You are welcome to our ward.'

The latter is shorter but is impersonal and emphasises the 'us' and 'them' that you are trying to avoid with patient involvement.

The content of any leaflet should be developed in conjunction with the rest of the team and most importantly with patients. Find out what it is that patients want to know before writing patient information. Remember that when giving patients written information it is good practice to explain the contents to them and check their understanding.

Patient feedback

Patient feedback

There are a number of ways of gaining feedback from patients, these include:

- surveys
- focus groups
- open surgeries
- exit cards
- suggestion boxes
- one-off forums
- telephone interviews
- patient diaries.

Each method has its disadvantages and advantages (see Table 8.1) and should be used according to the needs of the service.

Table 8.1   **Methods of getting patient feedback**

Method	Advantages	Disadvantages
surveys	relatively cheap and easily managed time efficient once the survey has been designed and an appropriate mailing list identified, it can be repeated easily	low response rates limited in scope unlikely to be completed by people who have low levels of literacy or for whom English is not their first language postage costs the issues focused on may not lead to areas of concern experienced by the patient difficult to express dis-satisfaction through a survey costly to analyse requires separate feedback to respondents
focus groups	can influence policy can be more powerful than staff opinion participants may offer resources free of charge will ensure patient-centred approach encourage discussion	can be time-consuming representatives may need training small number of people involved need skilled facilitation
open surgeries	easily accessible to patients and relatives do not need too much preparation	need skilled facilitation
exit cards	cheap and easily managed anonymity ensures honest feedback can be used continuously	easily forgotten not good for those with literacy problems
suggestion boxes	cheap and easily organised anonymity ensures honest feedback	easily forgotten not good for those with literacy problems
one-off forums	can be used continuously can influence policy	need skilled facilitation

one-off forums *(continued)*	can be more powerful than staff opinion participants may offer resources free of charge will ensure patient-centred approach	
telephone interviews	do not need dedicated space good for picking up extra information use of an independent person can protect anonymity and encourage views to be shared	fears about confidentiality poor quality data if people called when they are busy or preoccupied can be hard to reach people unable to offer support if the patient becomes emotional
involving patients in ward meetings	allows patients to have more influence with regard to specific services can increase sense of ownership informs the understanding and decision-making of the nurses in the meeting	patients may be seen as a 'token' presence only some patients will feel confident enough to take part in this way support needs can be time-consuming
patient diaries	can include facts, feelings and emotions can focus on the whole or part of the journey are relatively cheap will help the patient remember events	patients need to remember to complete them confidentiality can be an issue need time and commitment may produce a lot of information that may be difficult to analyse

To get patients' and relatives' immediate reaction to the care that they have received you could use a suggestion box or exit cards like this one:

JONES WARD

Please answer these three questions about your experience on Jones Ward. Your comments are taken very seriously and changes are made to the way we work wherever possible.

1. What did you like best about the Jones Ward?

2. What did you like least about Jones Ward?

3. What is the one thing you would change about the ward if you could?

Surveys are useful to get more detailed feedback or you can target specific topics such as staff attitude or the quality of care.

Focus groups are a good approach to use if you want to encourage discussion about a wide range of topics and they can be used effectively to influence decision making. They are informal and are usually made up of people with common characteristics, for example they may be people of the same age or with the same condition. You will need to consider how you will recruit partici-pants, where you will hold the meetings and the arrangements for access and refreshments (Modernisation Agency, 2005). Good facilitation is important to keep the discussion on track and to support participants who may find the discussion emotional.

Open surgeries are an informal approach that you can use in out-patient departments or on wards. Two people are needed to facilitate the session and it is useful if one person is a senior person working in the area. The surgery is held on site at a time when patients are available to come and talk to the facilitators, perhaps they are waiting for an appointment or at visiting times. They are encouraged to 'pop in' and chat to the facilitators about their experiences.

Patient diaries are used when you want to analyse the detail of the patient's view of the service. A diary does not need to be a written diary. It could be a video or tape recorder. Children might find it useful to draw pictures of their experience. You will need to make sure the patient understands what is expected of them. They may also need support when completing the diary and you may be able to address some of the issues as they arise.

Telephone interviews are a useful approach if you want to get feedback after the patient has been discharged. Prepare the questions in advance and make sure you get the patients' consent by writing to them in advance. It is not good practice to cold call. When you phone them check that they are still willing to participate and that the time is convenient.

Feedback to patients

Patient involvement is a two-way process. If you ask patients for their opinion you must feed back to them about the changes you have made. You will need to think about how you will achieve this, particularly if the suggestions or opinions are anonymous. If you have the patient's details you can write to them or invite them to a meeting to hear what has happened. Supermarkets and banks use noticeboards to tell customers what changes they have made as a result of the surveys they have carried out and this could easily be adopted in ward and department areas.

Dos and don'ts of patient involvement

Patient involvement

Before choosing a method of patient involvement consider what it is that you want to achieve. Don't patronise patients or use them as the token representative. Don't ask for their opinion if you don't intend to make any changes. Involve your team in obtaining patient feedback and then they will be more willing to take on board the suggestions for improvement. Get approval from your manager or the budget holder for what you are doing so that you have more leverage when asking for additional resources.

Don't expect patients to attend focus groups without paying them travel and car parking expenses. Provide feedback to staff about their interpersonal skills (see Chapter 5) to ensure that patients receive a courteous service. Don't tolerate staff being rude to patients. Explain all the care options to patients but don't use jargon or be too technical. Give patients time to communicate their needs. Involve patients and carers in discharge planning and assessment.

Remember that not all feedback will be positive. When it is negative, don't take it personally – do something about it.

Chapter 9
Measuring performance

Performance measurements are an important part of performance management (see Chapter 5). They are about having measurable objectives that can help you monitor progress and bring about improvement. They enable you to compare actual results with planned results. They help you define the information or data that you need to collect and demonstrate improvement in the service you provide.

Performance measurements are used by organisations to demonstrate improvement and progress. They are not just used in healthcare but are also used in industry. British Telecom uses the following indicators:

● percentage of women, ethnic minority and disabilities amongst employees

● lost time injury rate

● sickness absence rate

● ethical trading

● community contribution

● completion of training by employees.

BT's customer care measure shows how they use it to demonstrate their improvement in customer service. From 2003–2005 their objective was to reduce the number of dissatisfied customers by 25% a year for three years. The target for 2006 was to increase the number of 'extremely satisfied' and 'very satisfied' customers by 5%, thereby indicating their progress by moving customers' satisfaction from dissatisfied to extremely satisfied (www.btplc.com).

Performance targets

Performance targets

Performance targets have been a key element of the government's drive to improve the effectiveness of the NHS. They were first introduced as part of the NHS Plan in 2000 and the first targets were implemented in 2001. Table 9.1 demonstrates how some of targets have progressed since then.

Table 9.1

Development of Department of Health Targets since 2001

2001	2002	2003	2004
A reduction of the time patients wait for an in-patient appointment	A reduction in the number of patients waiting more than 18 months for an in-patient appointment	A reduction in the number of patients waiting more than 15 months for an in-patient appointment	A reduction in the number of patients waiting more than 12 months for an in-patient appointment
A reduction in the time patients wait for an out-patient appointment	A reduction in the number of patients waiting more than 26 weeks for an appointment	A reduction in the number of patients waiting more than 21 weeks for an appointment	A reduction in the number of patients waiting more than 17 weeks for an appointment
A reduction of the number of people with breast cancer waiting for more than 2 weeks for an appointment to see a specialist	A reduction of the number of people with cancer waiting for more than 2 weeks for an appointment to see a specialist	A reduction of the number of people with cancer waiting for more than 2 weeks for an appointment to see a specialist	A reduction of the number of people with cancer waiting for more than 2 weeks for an appointment to see a specialist

The NHS in England has focused performance measures in four areas.

Capacity and capability

These measures look at trust resources, how well the organisation is run, how staff are treated, working conditions and record keeping.

Key targets

These are the main determiners of the star ratings and include essential measures such as cancer and A&E waiting times.

Patient focus

Patient-focused measures are usually based on the results of patient surveys and demonstrate how well patients are being dealt with.

Clinical focus

These demonstrate the standard of treatment given and therefore the outcomes of treatment, such as mortality and readmission rates.

Each year the targets have become tighter and have introduced a 'softer' focus, introducing aspects of patient choice and improving staff experiences. *Standards for Better Health* (DH, 2004g) includes the following targets:

- patients will be able to choose from four to five providers for planned hospital care from December 2005
- by 2008, patients will have the right to choose from any healthcare provider which meets the Healthcare Commission's standards and which can provide the care within the price that the NHS will pay
- patients will be given more access to a wider range of services in primary care
- patient choice will be supported by the provision of information about waiting times at different providers and about the quality of care available
- there will be continuing increases in frontline NHS staff where these are required to meet patients' needs
- staff will be supported in working differently to make the best use of skills. For example, primary physicians and other practitioners with special interests will be enabled to deliver care more flexibly
- staff will be supported to fulfil their potential with the NHS Institute for Innovation and Improvement (NHSIII) and Skills Escalator helping staff develop throughout their careers
- extra pay for staff and pay linked to performance will create stronger incentives to deliver personalised care.

The government uses targets on a national basis to improve performance and monitor progress of trusts. Within trusts the targets are disseminated to departments and directorates for implementation.

Whilst the targets have put NHS staff under enormous pressure, there is no doubting that many, if not all, have had an enormous impact on the service the patient receives. It is no longer the norm to sit in Accident and Emergency waiting rooms for hours on end or to wait months for an out-patient appointment. Whatever we think of the targets they have helped the NHS maintain a focus and that is what performance measures are about. They are to give us something to focus on in order to improve the service we provide.

Why measure your team's performance?

National drivers

There are a number of national drivers for implementing performance measures in clinical teams.

The NHS Plan

The NHS Plan stated that the government would set standards of performance, monitor performance and set up a system for inspection in order to drive up standards of care. It announced the implementation of a Performance framework for all NHS Trusts. It said:

> *The NHS is an organisation glued together by a bond of trust between staff and patient or, what some have called 'principled motivation'. Our aim is to renew that for today's world, not throwing away those values to market mechanisms, but harnessing them to drive up performance.*

(DH, 2000)

Payment by Results

Payment by Results is a system of payment to trusts for the work they undertake. Payments will be made by Primary Care Trusts who will commission services on the basis of case mix and the number of treatment episodes. The prices are based on a national tariff which standardises prices nationally with regional variations for wages and the cost of delivery. The implication for organisations and teams is that they will need to demonstrate cost effectiveness.

Choice

In 2003, the DH published *Building on the Best* which sets out the patient choice agenda. The principle is to empower patients, enabling them to make choices about their healthcare. This ranges from ensuring they have access to information to being able to

The NHS plan

Payment by results

Choice

choose which hospital they go to for their treatment. This introduces competition to trusts who will have to demonstrate that they deliver high standards of care in order to attract patients to their service. For clinical teams this means that demonstrating performance is essential.

National Service Frameworks

National Service Frameworks

National Service Frameworks are long-term strategies for improving areas of care. There are frameworks for coronary heart disease, cancer, paediatric intensive care, older people, diabetes, long-term conditions, and renal services. The frameworks set standards and lay out strategies to support their implementation. Their purpose is to raise quality of care and reduce variation by setting out national plans that are translated into local practice.

Local drivers

Local drivers

From a local perspective the drivers for measuring your performance are:

- the need to improve patient care
- the need to reduce variation in practice
- cost effectiveness
- the need to show that care is safe, timely, beneficial, compassionate, patient-centred, equitable and efficient
- to determine whether the level of care is of an acceptable standard.

There is also a wealth of evidence that suggests that measuring performance benefits the team by increasing motivation and retention. Patient-centred measures also help to keep the focus of the team on what's best for the patient (ICN, 2005).

Traditionally, medical care has been measured by death, disease, disability and disability rates. Florence Nightingale used mortality statistics as a quality of care measure for British soldiers during the Crimean War. We now need to be more sophisticated about what we measure in order to meet patients' increasing needs.

The information obtained from using indicators can be used to develop services as they will help to identify areas of the service that need improving. It will help you and your team to reflect on practice and its impact on patients. It will also help to share clinical knowledge and encourage learning.

Improving patient outcomes

Nursing has long struggled to express its value. Try thinking about your practice in terms of interventions and the outcomes those interventions have. Are the patients in your care better off because of what you do? It sounds simplistic, but can you demonstrate that they are? Some simple questions you can ask yourself and your team are:

- do the patients in my care have fewer symptoms as a result of what I do?
- do the patients in my care understand what they need to do to maintain their health?
- will patients in my care be able to cope better at home because of my intervention?
- what are the effects of my interventions on each patient I have contact with?

(Oermann, 1999)

The difficulty with measuring the nursing impact on patient care is separating the nurse's input from the multi-disciplinary input.

Problems with performance measures

Performance measures

Measuring the impact of nursing on patient outcomes is complex as it can be difficult to show a cause and effect relationship between what nurses do, as opposed to what other members of the team do, for the patient.

Performance measures are not without their pitfalls and can be misinterpreted or manipulated. There have been anecdotal examples with government targets: patients being moved round the corner from A&E departments so as not to breach the four-hour target; and patients being moved to inappropriate beds for the same reason. A performance measure should be clearly defined to avoid distortion of clinical priorities or provide 'perverse' incentives. It can also be difficult to evaluate the input of one professional in a multi-disciplinary team.

Performance measures can increase stress for already overworked staff, which makes it extremely important that they understand why the measures are in place and how they have been reached. Finally, performance measures and targets should not be used to punish or blame people. They should be used as a learning tool if targets are not reached and a reward when they are.

Getting started

Performance measures must be used to support your objectives and your overall mission, vision or philosophy (see Chapter 6). They have to be realistic (you don't want to set yourself up to fail) and they should be measurable. If you choose something where the supporting data is already being collected you will save yourself a lot of time, but you shouldn't shirk away from something that needs measuring.

Firstly, identify what it is you want to measure and what your priorities are for your patients and your team. To help you decide what to measure consider the following:

incident and accident forms – is there an area of concern?

patient concerns/complaints – is there an issue that patients consistently report?

risk assessments and audits – are risk assessments being carried out?

Essence of Care benchmarking – has it highlighted an area of poor practice?

compliments – is there something that your team is really good at?

new practice – are you doing something different that would be good to share?

directorate and trust priorities.

If you want to focus on nursing make sure that the measures are within the responsibilities of the role and that the practice is evidence-based. It should also be developed from the patients' perspective so you need to involve them in the process (see Chapter 8).

Remember that you want to improve practice but you can also use performance measurement to demonstrate your success. A mixture of the two is ideal for maintaining staff morale and motivation. When you have decided what you want to measure you need to develop it into an 'indicator'. This is the term used for the particular measurement. It acts as a trigger to alert you to any problems there may be with your team's performance and it should be valid and reliable.

Types of indicator

Types of indicator

There are three types of indicator, according to Avedis Donabedian (Donabedian, 1980).

Structure indicators
Structure indicators measure the environment in which healthcare is provided. They are about *having* the right things.

Some examples are staffing (for example, the number of registered nurse hours per patient per day), staff training, team organisation, policies and protocols, equipment and buildings.

Process indicators
Process indicators measure the method by which care is provided. They are about *doing* the right things.

Some examples are the use of risk assessments, treatments, staff satisfaction (as this impacts on patient outcomes) and the use of care pathways.

Outcome indicators
Outcome indicators reflect what happens to a patient after an intervention has been carried out or not carried out. They are about the right things *happening*.

Some examples are infection rates, pressure sore incidents, patient satisfaction and mortality rates.

Generally process and structure indicators tend to be easier to measure and outcome measures are best for assessing quality. Ideally you should use all three (see Table 9.2).

Table 9.2

Types of indicator

Structure	Process	Outcome
Hand-washing protocol developed and distributed to all wards and departments	Proportion of staff washing hands	Number of incidents of hospital-acquired MRSA
Number of PDRS training sessions available for line managers to attend	Number of managers attending PDRS training	Number of staff receiving annual PDRS
Provision of education for patients to support self-care	Number of patients receiving education	Proportion of patients enabled to self-care

As discussed previously, it can be extremely difficult to demonstrate a cause and effect relationship between nursing care and patient outcomes. Doran defines nursing sensitive indicators as:

> *outcomes for which the individual nurse can be held accountable ... relevant, based on nurses' scope and domain of practice and for which there is empirical evidence linking nursing inputs and interventions to the outcome.*

(Doran, 2003)

There are a number of structure and process factors for which there is empirical evidence linking nursing inputs and interventions to a positive impact on patient care. By measuring these you will demonstrate good management practices and be contributing to better patient outcomes. These include staffing levels, skill mix, team working, shift patterns and the organisation of nursing.

Table 9.3 shows some of the things you might want to measure. Be careful not to lift these straight from the book and implement them. You need to get your staff and patients involved first. Patient involvement will help you ensure that you are meeting patients' expectations.

The indicator should also be understood by those who are trying to achieve it. Keep it simple and it will be easier to report and more easily understood by everyone. You might be sharing the information with patients and carers as well as staff and so it is best to avoid jargon. If the measures you are using reflect national policies, make sure that your definitions are the same. This will help you benchmark with other organisations and with national figures.

Remember to check for perverse incentives. An example of this occurred in call centres where staff were expected to answer a number of calls within a certain timeframe, which they achieved by picking up the phone and immediately putting it down! The target was met but customer satisfaction plummeted.

Indicators can be measured quantitatively or qualitatively. Quantitative measures answer questions such as 'how many?', 'how much?' and 'what percentage?'. You might collect quantitative data by auditing patients' notes or simply by reviewing staff rotas. Qualitative measures are subjective and therefore the data collection methods will be different. You may want to hold focus groups or undertake staff satisfaction surveys. Qualitative

Improving patient outcomes

Table 9.3   **Suggested indicators**

Topic	Examples
Staff sickness	number of days lost to sickness per month number of sick days as a percentage of working days
Staff turnover	percentage rate of staff turnover*
Skill mix	ratio of qualified nurses to unqualified nurses
Staff uptake of mandatory training	percentage of staff who attend manual handling training
Tissue viability	number of patients with a hospital-acquired pressure ulcer as a percentage of the patient population percentage of patients who receive a Waterlow Pressure Ulcer Risk Assessment
Complaints	number of complaints relating to staff attitude as a percentage of total complaints
Readmission rates	number of patients readmitted within 30 days of discharge
Incidents	number of drug administration incidents per month
Patient education	percentage of patients receiving written and verbal information during their hospital stay
Urinary tract infections	the number of patients with a hospital-acquired urinary tract infection as a percentage of the patient population
Discharge planning	number of discharge plans completed within two days of admission number of community staff notified of patient discharge two days prior to discharge date
Drug administration	number of interruptions during drug rounds
Leg ulcers	percentage of leg ulcers treated by nurses only which healed within 6 months of treatment starting
Pain	percentage of patients reporting lower pain scores due to new intervention
Infection rates in cannula sites	number of infections as a percentage of the number of patients with cannulas inserted
Patient falls	the number of falls of all patients as a percentage of all patients

measures are just as important and again you may choose to have a combination of both. The indicators should either address an area of poor practice or concern that you want to improve or demonstrate an area of practice that you know you are good at. Again, a combination of both is ideal.

Once you have determined your measure or indicator you will need to define the terms to enable comparisons to be made. For example, if you were using the process indicator:

discharge plan completed within two days of admission

you would need to define whose discharge plans count towards this indicator – all patients, just patients with a certain condition or patients over a certain age. Does it matter who has completed the discharge plan and what do you mean by completed (remember the perverse incentives)? Also, define which area you are in and consider what will happen to your data at bank holidays and weekends.

Next you will need to be clear about why you are using this particular measure. This particularly needs to be transparent to those who will be collecting the data or those who are under extra pressure as a result of the measure. Equally your manager may want to know why you are using that target instead of one that would be more relevant to them.

You will also need to establish your baseline. Using the same example, how many discharge plans are currently completed within two days of admission? If the answer is none then you have a lot more work to do than if your current baseline is 75% but it may be important that the work is done.

You have now identified the:

- indicator
- definition
- rationale
- baseline.

Demonstrating progress

No matter what your baseline you will want to demonstrate that your service delivery or quality of care has improved. In order to demonstrate your progress you will need to set targets, for example:

Number of discharge plans completed within two days of admission is currently 49%.

Target for next six months is 75%.

With each measure, consider what the desirable level is. For example, if your measure is related to pain the tolerance will be much less:

100% patients to have their pain levels assessed and medication administered according to protocol.

Set realistic targets and once you have achieved them set new targets.

Getting your team involved

Getting your team involved

Implementing performance measures will in itself help to motivate your team. To ensure their commitment you should involve as many members as possible in the development of the indicators. You will be relying on team members to change their practice and to collect data. Without their involvement you will not succeed. Chapter 2 explains more about the process of change.

Make sure that all the members of the team understand your expectations. It may be difficult to measure individuals' influence on the improvement of team performance as a whole. At the outset you need to be clear about their roles and responsibilities in relation to each measure.

Include performance measures in staff appraisals to ensure that everyone is focused on them and that individuals are given the training they need to change their practice. If you have been successful ensure people are praised individually. Think about how you will reward the team.

If measuring the team's performance shows that they are not performing as well as expected, identify the causes, discuss them with the team and look for possible solutions. Above all, avoid blame. Use the situation to help the team develop their performance.

Data

Data

The data you collect must be reliable and, perhaps most importantly, believed by your team. If you know, for example, that the number of incident forms that you complete reporting patient falls exceeds the number being fed back to you in organisational reports then you need to challenge the data.

Check whether the data is already being collected. Your manager may know or you could try contacting other people within your organisation such as clinical governance, finance, human resources and service development. Find out how often it is collected as this will influence how often you measure the target. If the data is not currently being collected you will need to consider how you are going to gather the information you need.

When you have the information you need think about how you are going to report your data to show your improvement. Your trust may already have a format and where possible you should adopt this. Figure 9.1 gives some examples:

Figure 9.1

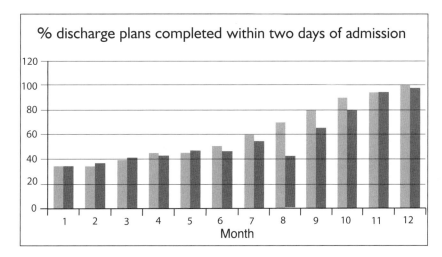

% discharge plans completed within two days of admission											
Jan	Feb	Mar	Apr	May	June	July	Aug	Sept	Oct	Nov	Dec
35	35	40	45	45	50	60	70	80	90	95	100
(35)	(37)	(42)	(43)	(48)	(48)	(55)	(43)	(65)	(80)	(95)	(98)

Numbers without brackets indicate target. Numbers with brackets indicate actual figure.

% discharge plans completed within two days of admission

Or you simply might want to report the figures in writing. Think of your audience and choose an appropriate format accordingly. You may need to use a different format for different audiences.

When considering whom to share your results with, think about your 'WIIFMs' or 'What's in it for me?' You will naturally tell your team and your manager, but if you've done well don't be afraid to tell the world! What about sharing the data with other areas and the hierarchy within your organisation? Consider:

- your peers
- the director of nursing
- the trust board
- commissioners
- the strategic health authority
- primary care trusts/acute trusts
- patient carer groups
- journals
- conferences
- national groups.

You will not be likely to be able to demonstrate positive progress immediately but your performance measures will help you identify where you need to improve. Don't be afraid to discuss the results with your team in order to find out why you haven't performed well but be careful to do this in a non-punitive fashion. You need to find out where you can improve and you can only do this if your team is open and honest.

The positive information that you have gathered from measuring your performance can also be used for staff recruitment. Information that shows that you need more resources can be used to support requests for an increase in your budget and should be used in conjunction with the business planning cycle.

By including performance measures in staff appraisals you will ensure that everyone is focused on them. If you have been successful you can ensure people are praised individually.

Figure 9.2 below shows the stages of implementing performance measures

Figure 9.2   **The stages of implementing performance measures**

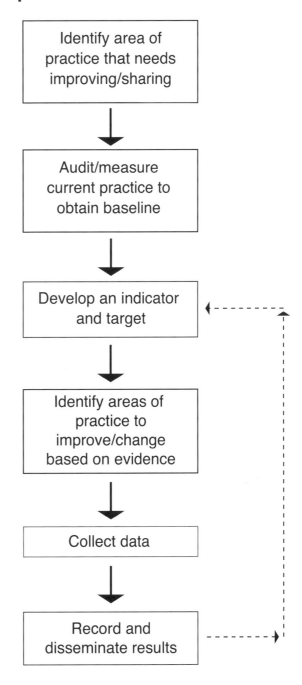

Appendix 1
Interview scoring template

Name of applicant   Job title applied for

Interviewer   Date

Instructions: Carefully evaluate applicant's interview performance against your questions. Assign points (0–3) for each category. Points should then be totalled and averaged to give an overall interview score.

0 = insufficient evidence   1 = poor evidence   2 = satisfactory evidence   3 = good evidence

Competence	Question(s)	Keywords	Comments	Score
Experience				
Education				
Communication skills				
Professional knowledge				

Appendix 2
Team work survey

Objectives

To identify the stage of the team work model that your team is presently operating in.

Instructions

This questionnaire contains statements about team work. Next to each statement, indicate how often your team displays each behaviour by using the following scoring system:

- almost never – 1
- seldom – 2
- occasionally – 3
- frequently – 4
- almost always – 5

1.	We try to have set procedures or protocols to ensure that things are orderly and run smoothly (e.g. minimise interruptions so that everyone gets the opportunity to have their say).	
2.	We are quick to get on with the task on hand and do not spend too much time in the planning stage.	
3.	Our team feels that we are all in it together and shares responsibilities for the team's success or failure.	
4.	We have thorough procedures for agreeing on our objectives and planning the way we will perform our tasks.	
5.	Team members are afraid or do not like to ask others for help.	
6.	We take our team's goals and objectives literally, and assume a shared understanding.	
7.	The team leader tries to keep order and contributes to the task in hand.	
8.	We do not have fixed procedures. We make them up as the task or project progresses.	
9.	We generate lots of ideas but we do not use many of them because we fail to listen to them and reject them without fully understanding them.	
10.	Team members do not fully trust the other members and closely monitor others who are working on a specific task.	

11.	The team leader ensures that we follow the procedures, do not argue, do not interrupt and keep to the point.
12.	We enjoy working together. We have a fun and productive time.
13.	We have accepted each other as members of the team.
14.	The team leader is democratic and collaborative.
15.	We are trying to define the goal and what tasks need to be accomplished.
16.	Many of the team members have their own ideas about the process and personal agendas are rampant.
17.	We fully accept each other's strengths and weakness.
18.	We assign specific roles to team members (team leader, facilitator, time keeper, note taker and so on).
19.	We try to achieve harmony by avoiding conflict.
20.	The tasks are very different to what we imagined and seem very difficult to accomplish.
21.	There are many abstract discussions of the concepts and issues, which make some members impatient.
22.	We are able to work through group problems.
23.	We argue a lot even though we agree on the real issues.
24.	The team is often tempted to go beyond the original scope of the project.
25.	We express criticism of others constructively.
26.	There is a close attachment to the team.
27.	It seems as if little is being accomplished with the project's goals.
28.	The goals we have established seem unrealistic.
29.	Although we are not fully sure of the project's goals and issues, we are excited and proud to be on the team.
30.	We often share personal problems with each other.
31.	There is a lot of resistance to the tasks in hand and quality improvement approaches.
32.	We get a lot of work done.

Scoring

Next to each statement number below, transfer the score that you gave that statement on the questionnaire. For example, if you scored statement one with a 3 (occasionally), then enter a 3 next to item one below. When you have entered all the scores for each statement, total each of the four columns.

Item score	Item score	Item score	Item score
1. _____	2. _____	4. _____	3. _____
5. _____	7. _____	6. _____	8. _____
10. _____	9. _____	11. _____	12. _____
15. _____	16. _____	13. _____	14. _____
18. _____	20. _____	19. _____	17. _____
21. _____	23. _____	24. _____	22. _____
27. _____	28. _____	25. _____	26. _____
29. _____	31. _____	30. _____	32. _____
TOTAL _____	TOTAL _____	TOTAL _____	TOTAL _____
Forming stage	Storming stage	Normingstage	Performing stage

This questionnaire is to help you assess at what stage your team normally operates. It is based on the Tuckman model of Forming, Storming, Norming, and Performing. The lowest score possible for a stage is 8 (almost never), while the highest score possible for a stage is 40 (almost always).

The highest of the four scores indicates which stage you perceive your team to normally operates in. If your highest score is 32 or more, it is a strong indicator of the stage your team is in.

The lowest of the three scores is an indicator of the stage your team is furthest away from. If your lowest score is 16 or less, it is a strong indicator that your team does not operate this way.

If two of the scores are close to the same, you are probably going through a transitional phase, except:

● if you score highly in both the Forming and Storming stages then you are in the Storming stage

● if you score highly in both the Norming and Performing stages then you are in the Performing stage.

If there is only a small difference between three or four scores, then this indicates that: you have no clear perception of the way your team operates; the team's performance is highly variable; or that you are in the Storming stage (this stage can be extremely volatile with high and low points).

Improving patient outcomes

Reliability and validity

Since this survey is a training tool, it has not been formally checked for reliability or validity. However, on the basis of feedback from various sources, I believe that it is fairly accurate.

Appendix 3
Providing references

You are not under any legal obligation to give a reference for an employee unless it states that this is an expectation in the contract of employment. It is, however, considered a moral obligation, particularly if an offer of employment will only be given if you provide a reference.

Any reference you give should be factual and should describe employment history, qualifications, and experience. If you don't have the facts and are unable to obtain them, then say so in the reference. If you are giving information about the individual's sickness record you should first ensure that they are aware you are giving that information, and if you are giving details about their medical conditions you need their permission to do so.

It is good practice to discuss your reference with the individual and poor practice to include anything about their performance that you haven't had opportunity to discuss with them (see TSB plc v Harris below).

The legal position
There is no specific law that relates to writing references, but there is legislation which is relevant and you should be aware of.

● Unfair Contract Terms Act 1977 may apply to attempts to disclaim liability for a reference

● Data Protection Act 1998 may also apply to the processing of information in the provision of a reference

● Discrimination acts relating to sex, sexual orientation, religion or disability and age

There are a number of cases in law relating to references which include:

● TSB Bank plc v Harris [2000] IRLR 157

● Bartholomew v London Borough of Hackney [1999] IRLR 246

● Spring v Guardian Assurance PLC [1994] IRLR 460

The court in the Bartholomew v London Borough of Hackney said a reference 'must be in substance true, accurate and fair and must not give a misleading impression but it does have to be full and comprehensive'.

In the case of Spring v Guardian Assurance plc [1994] IRLR 460, the court found that the employer providing the reference might be liable for any damages if the employee suffers any economic loss as a result of a negligent mis-statement.

The case of TSB plc v Harris was brought because TSB had written a reference about Ms Harris which said that there had been 19 customer complaints about her. This was factual but Ms Harris was only aware of two complaints. The court therefore upheld Ms Harris's claim of unfair dismissal. It said:

> It is a breach of trust and confidence to disclose complaints to others which the employee has not had the opportunity to answer.

You should also be aware that under the Data Protection Act 1998 an employee can ask their new employer for a copy of the reference even if you have specified that the reference is confidential. It is considered good practice for the new employer to seek the author's consent, but for your own protection you should ensure that the reference is 'true, accurate and fair'.

Appendix 4
Templates for effective meetings

Terms of reference template

[Title of meeting]
Terms of reference

Purpose of the meeting
Frequency of meetings
Participants
Attendance at meetings
Dates and times of meetings
Venue
Note keeping
Ground rules
Setting the agenda
Chairing

Improving patient outcomes

Minutes template

[Title of meeting]

Minutes

[Date]

In attendance	Apologies
Chairperson	

Notes	Lead
Agenda item 1	
Agenda item 2	
Agenda item 3	
Agenda item 4	
Date and time of next meeting	

Appendices

Action notes template

[Title of meeting]

Action notes

[Date]

In attendance	Apologies
Chairperson	

Action	Timescales	Lead
Date and time of next meeting		

Improving patient outcomes

Appendix 5
Return to work interview template

Return to Work – Interview Form	
Name	
Job title	
Ward/Department	
First day of absence	
Last day of absence	
Total number of days absent	
Is absence due to injury at work?	

What was the cause of illness? Did you need to seek doctor's or hospital attention?

Have you suffered from this type of illness in the past year?
If so please state when and how long it lasted (approx).

Do you feel that you have fully recovered from your illness to return to work?
Is there anything else you would like to tell me which is affecting your recovery or the likelihood of this illness happening again?

Do you feel that there is anything we can do to support you?

Proposed course of action (including referral to occupational health or human resources)

Manager's signature	Date
Employee's signature	Date

Appendix 6
Complaints analysis pro forma

Date complaint received	Details of complaint	Subject matter	Action taken	Date response sent/resolved

Common acronyms

ACAS	Advisory Conciliation and Arbitration Service
BMA	British Medical Association
CIPD	Chartered Institute of Personnel and Development
CGST	Clinical Governance Support Team
DH	Department of Health
DWP	Department of Work and Pensions
ICN	International Council of Nurses
HSCIC	Health and Social Care Information Centre
NAO	National Audit Office
NCCSDO	National Coordinating Centre for NHS Service Delivery and Organisation Research and Development
NCEPOD	National Confidential Enquiry into Perioperative Deaths
NHS	National Health Service
NHSIII	NHS Institute for Innovation and Improvement
NHSME	NHS Management Executive
NHSRU	National Health Service Research Unit
NMC	Nursing and Midwifery Council
NPSA	National Patient Safety Agency
PALS	Patient Advice and Liaison Service
RCN	Royal College of Nursing
SCOPME	The Standing Committee on Postgraduate Medical and Dental Education

References

ACAS (2004) *Tackling Discrimination and Promoting Equality – Good Practice Guide for Employers* London: ACAS.

ACAS (2005) *Absence and Labour Turnover Advisory Booklet* London: ACAS.

Aggleton, P. and Chalmers, H. (2000) *Nursing Models and Nursing Practice* Hampshire: Palgrave Macmillan.

Aiken, L.H., Clarke, S.P., Sloane, D.M., Sochalski, J. and Silber J.H. (2002) Hospital nurse staffing and patient mortality, nurse burnout, and job dissatisfaction. *Journal of the American Medical Association* 288: 1987–1993.

Allen, I. (2001) *Stress among Ward Sisters and Charge Nurses*. London: Policy Studies Institute.

Ambrose, C. (2002) Recruitment problems in intensive care: a solution. *Nursing Standard* 17(12).

Baker, L. (2005) Recruiting and training senior nurses using a rotational model. *Nursing Times* 101(12).

Bauman, A., Fardy, J., Harris, P. (2003) Getting it right: why bother with patient centred care? *Medical Journal of Australia* 179(5): 253–256.

Beagrie, S. (2004) Assessment centres: how to cut it at assessment centres. *Personnel Today* 5 October.

Beckford-Ball, J. (2005) How to improve the safety of patients treated in the NHS. *Nursing Times* 101(49).

Bergquist, W. (1993) *The Modern Organization: Mastering the Art of Irreversible Change*. San Francisco: Jossey-Bass.

Binnie, A. and Titchen, A. (1998) *Freedom to Practice: A Study of the Development of Patient Centred Nursing in an Acute Medical Unit* London: RCN.

Binnie, A. and Titchen, A. (1999) *Freedom to Practice: The Development of Patient Centred Nursing* Oxford: Butterworth Heinemann.

Bird, D. (2005) Patient safety: improving incident reporting. *Nursing Standard* 20(14–15–16): 43–46.

BMA (2004) *Dealing with Discrimination: Guidelines for BMA Members* London: BMA.

BMA (2005) *Safe Handover: Safe Patients* London: BMA.

Borrill, C.S., Carletta, J., Carter, A.J., Dawson, J.F., Garrod, S., Rees, A., Richards, A., Shapiro, D., and West, M. A. (2001) *The Effectiveness of Health Care Teams in the National Health Service* (Final report from the project 'Health Care Team Composition and Functioning as Determinants of Effectiveness', 121/6302) Leeds: DH.

Borrill, C. and West, M. (2001) *Developing Team Working in Healthcare* Birmingham: Aston University.

Bradshaw, P. (2003) Ethics, power and policy – the future of nursing in the NHS. *Journal of Nursing Management* 11(5): 360.

Brearly, S. (1990) *Patient Participation: The Literature* Harrow: Scutari Press.

Bridges, W. and Bridges, S.M. (2000) Leading transition: a new model for change. *Leader to Leader* 16: 30–36.

Buchan, J., Ball, J. and Rafferty, A.M. (2003) *A Lasting Attraction? The 'Magnet' Accreditation of Rochdale Infirmary* London: London School of Hygiene and Tropical Medicine.

Buchan, J., Thompson, M. and O'May, F. (2000) *Incentive and remuneration strategies. Health workforce incentive and remuneration. A research review.* Discussion paper 4 Geneva: WHO.

Byrne, M.W. and Keefe, M.R. (2002) Building research competence in nursing through mentoring. *Journal of Nursing Scholarship* 34(4): 391–396.

CGST (2005) *A Practical Handbook For Clinical Audit* London: DH.

CIPD (2005) CIPD website: www.cipd.co.uk.

CIPD (2005a) *Recruitment, Retention, and Turnover Annual Survey Report* London: CIPD.

CIPD (2005b) *Performance Management Survey Report* London: CIPD.

Clarke, S.P., Sloane, D.M. and Aiken, L.H. (2002) Effects of hospital staffing and organizational climate on needlestick injuries to nurses. *American Journal of Public Health* 92(7):1115–1119.

Clifford, C. (2004) *Getting Research into Practice* Edinburgh: Churchill Livingstone.

Clutterbuck, D. (2004) *Everyone Needs a Mentor* London: CIPD.

Collins, M. (2006) Taking a lead on stress: rank and relationship awareness in the NHS. *Journal of Nursing Management* 14(4): 310–317.

Cork, A. (2005) A model for successful change management. *Nursing Standard* 19(25): 40–42.

Coulter, A. (2002) After Bristol: putting patients at the centre. *Quality and Safety in Healthcare* 11: 186–188.

Crookes, P.A. (2004) *Research into Practice: Essential Skills for Reading and Applying Research in Nursing and Healthcare*, 2nd edn, London: Baillière Tindall.

Cronin, S.N. (1999) Recognition of staff nurse job performance and achievements: staff manager perceptions. *Journal of Nursing Administration* 29(1): 26–319.

Currie, V., Harvey, G., West, E., McKenna, H. and Keeney, S. (2005) Relationship between quality of care, staffing levels, skill mix and nurse autonomy: literature review. *Journal of Advanced Nursing* 51(1): 73–82.

Davies, S. and Priestley, M.J. (2006) A reflective evaluation of patient handover practices. *Nursing Standard* 20(21): 49–52.

Dawson, J., Taylor-Whilde, E. and Torkington, S. (2001) *Clinical Effectiveness in Nursing Practice* Philadelphia: Whurr Publishing.

Deegan, C., Watson, A., Nestor, G., Conlon, C. and Connaughton, F. (2005) Managing change initiatives in clinical areas. *Nursing Management (Harrow)* 12(4): 24–29.

Deming, W.E. (1989) *Out of the Crisis* Cambridge, MA: MIT.

DH (1989) *Working for Patients* London: HMSO.

DH (1991) *The Patient's Charter* London: HMSO.

DH (2000) *An Organisation with a Memory* London: The Stationery Office.

DH (2000a) *The NHS Plan* London: The Stationery Office.

DH (2001) *Learning from Bristol: the report of the public inquiry into children's heart surgery at the Bristol Royal Infirmary 1984–1995* London: The Stationery Office.

DH (2001a) *The Essence of Care: Patient-Focused Benchmarking for Healthcare Practitioners* London: The Stationery Office.

DH (2003a) *Building on the Best: Choice, Responsiveness and Equity in the NHS* London: The Stationery Office.

DH (2003b) *Strengthening Accountability: Involving Patients and the Public: Practice Guidance (Section 11 of The Health and Social Care Act 2001)* London: The Stationery Office.

DH (2004a) *The NHS Knowledge and Skills Framework (NHS KSF) and the Development Review Process* London: The Stationery Office.

DH (2004b) *Improving Working Lives Practice Plus National Audit Instrument* London: The Stationery Office.

DH (2004c) *Patient and Public Involvement in Health: The Evidence for Policy Implementation* London: The Stationery Office.

DH (2004d) *Practice Based Commissioning: Engaging Practices in Commissioning* London: The Stationery Office.

DH (2004e) *Financial Reforms – Payment by Results NHS Foundation Trusts Information Guide.* London: The Stationery Office.

DH (2004f) *Agenda for Change: What Will it Mean to You? A Guide for Staff* London: The Stationery Office.

DH (2004g) *Standards for Better Health* London: The Stationery Office.

DH (2005) *Now I Feel Tall – What a Patient Led NHS Feels Like* London: The Stationery Office.

DH (2006a) *Handling Concerns about the Performance of Healthcare Professionals: Principles of Good Practice* London: The Stationery Office.

DH (2006b) A Stronger Local Voice: A Framework for Creating a Stronger Local Voice in the Development of Health and Social Care London: The Stationery Office.

DH (2006c) *Our Health, Our Care, Our Say* London: The Stationery Office.

DH (forthcoming) *Implementation of Electronic Patient Handover* London: The Stationery Office.

Donabedian, A. (1980) *Explorations in Quality Assessment and Monitoring. 1. The Definition of Quality and Approaches to its Assessment* Chicago: Health Administration Press, American College of Healthcare Executives.

Doran, D.M. (ed.) (2003) *Nursing-Sensitive Outcomes: State of the Science* Massachusetts: Bartlett.

DWP (2005) *Focus on Older People* London: The Stationery Office.

Edell-Gustafsson, U. (2002) Sleep quality and responses to insufficient sleep in women on different work shifts. *Journal of Clinical Nursing* 11(2): 280–287.

Fitzpatrick, J., While, A. and Roberts, J. (1999) Shift work and its impact upon nurse performance: current knowledge and research issues. *Journal of Advanced Nursing* 29(1): 18–27.

Forsyth, S. and McKenzie, H. (2006) A comparative analysis of contemporary nurses' discontents. *Journal of Advanced Nursing* 56(2): 209–216.

Grantham, G., McMillan, V., Dunn, S., Gassner, A-L. and Woodcock, P. (2006) Patient self-medication – a change in hospital practice. *Journal of Clinical Nursing* 15(8): 962–970.

Gribben, R. (2004) Wrong candidates cost Britain £12bn. *Daily Telegraph* 21 June.

Gullick, J. (2004) The effect of an organisational model on the standard of care. *Nursing Times* 100(10): 36–9.

Hader, R. (2004) It's all in the way you say 'thanks'. *Nursing Management* 35(3): 4.

Healthcare Commission (2004) *The NHS Staff Survey*. London: Healthcare Commission.

Healthcare Commission (2005) *Acute Hospital Portfolio Review: Ward Staffing*. London: Healthcare Commission.

Hersey, P. and Blanchard, K.H. (1977) *The Management of Organizational Behaviour* New Jersey: Prentice Hall.

Honey, P. and Mumford, A. (1992) *Manual of Learning Styles* Maidenhead: Peter Honey

Hurst, K. (1993) *Nursing Workforce Planning* Harlow: Longman Information & Reference.

ICN (2000) *Nurses and Shift Work* Geneva: ICN.

ICN (2001) *It's Your Career: Take Charge, Career Planning and Development* Geneva: ICN.

ICN (2003) *Nurse:Patient Ratios* ICN Factsheet, available at www.icn.ch

ICN (2005) *What Makes a Good Employer* Geneva: ICN.

Iles, V. and Sutherland, K. (2001) *Managing Change in the NHS: Organisational Change: A Review for Healthcare Managers, Professionals and Researchers* London: NCCSDO.

Jick, T. D. (1991) *Implementing Change* Case Note 9: 191–114 Boston, MA: Harvard Business School Press.

Johnson, C.J., Croghan, E. and Crawford, J. (2003) The problem and management of sickness absence in the NHS: considerations for nurse managers. *Journal of Nursing Management* 11: 336–342.

Johnson, S. (1997) *Pathways of Care* Oxford: Blackwell Science.

Joshua-Amadi, M. (2003) Recruitment and retention in the NHS: a study in motivation. *Nursing Management* 9(9): 14–19.

Kangas, S., Kee, C. and McKee-Waddle, R. (1999) Organizational factors: nurses' job satisfaction and patient satisfaction with nursing care. *Journal of Nursing Administration* 29(1): 32–42.

Kay, D. and Hinds, R. (2002) *A Practical Guide to Mentoring* Oxford: How to books.

Kelly, M. (2005) Change from office-based to a walk-around handover system. *Nursing Times* 101(10): 34–35.

King's Fund (1988) *Research in Action: Developing the Role of the Ward Sister.* London: King's Fund Centre.

Kitson, A.L. (1991) *Therapeutic Nursing and the Hospitalised Elderly* London: Scutari Press.

Kotter, J.P. (1990) What leaders really do. In Mintzberg, H., Kotter, J. P. and Zaleznik, A. (eds) *Harvard Business Review: On Leadership* Boston MA: Harvard Business School Press.

Lister, S. (2006) NHS Sheds 2000 Jobs in a Week *The Times* 23 March.

Maben, J., Latter, S. and Clark, J. (2006) The theory-practice gap: impact of professional-bureaucratic work conflict on newly-qualified nurses. *Journal of Advanced Nursing* 55(4): 465–477.

Maccoby, M. (2003) The seventh rule: creating a learning culture. *Research Technology Management* 43(3): 59–60.

Madison, J. (1994) The value of mentoring in nursing leadership: a descriptive study. *Nursing Forum* 29(4): 16–23.

McCarty, G., Tyrell, M. and Cronin, C. (2002) *National Study of Turnover in Nursing and Midwifery* Dublin: Department of Health and Children.

McMahon, R. (1990) What are we saying? *Nursing Times* 86(25): 38–40.

Mehrabian, A. and Ferris, S.R. (1967) Inference of attitudes from nonverbal communication in two channels. *Journal of Consulting Psychology* 31: 248–252.

Modernisation Agency (2004) *Layers of Leadership: Hidden Influencers of Healthcare Improvement* London: Modernisation Agency.

Modernisation Agency (2005a) *Involving Patients and Carers* London: DH.

Modernisation Agency (2005b) *Process Mapping, Analysis and Redesign* London: DH.

Moroney, N. and Knowles, C. (2006) Innovation and teamwork: introducing multi-disciplinary team ward rounds. *Nursing Management* (Harrow) 13(1): 28–31.

Mohrman, S.A., Cohen, S.G. and Mohrman, A.M. Jr (1995) *Designing Team Based Organisations* San Francisco: Jossey-Bass.

NAO (2005) *A Safer Place for Patients* London: DH.

NCEPOD (2002) *Functioning as a Team? The 2002 Report* Available at www.ncepod.org.uk.

Nessling, R. (1990) *Manpower Monograph 2 – Skill Mix: A Practical Approach for Health Professionals* London: DH.

NHS Executive (1999) *Report of the Review of Nursing at Eastbourne Hospitals NHS Trust* London: The Stationery Office.

NHSIII (2005) *Lean Six Sigma* London: The Stationery Office.

NHSRU (2006) *Strategies and Outcomes Associated with Magnet Hospitals* Factsheet, available at www.nhsru.com.

Nightingale, F. (1859) *Notes on Nursing: What it is and what it is not* London: Heinemann.

NMC (2002) *Code of Professional Conduct* London: NMC.

NMC (2004) *Reporting Lack of Competence: A Guide for Employers and Managers* London: NMC.

NMC (2005) *Fitness to Practice* NMC Annual Report 2004–5. London: NMC.

NPSA (2004) *Seven Steps to Patient Safety: Your Guide to Safer Patient Care* London: The Stationery Office.

NPSA (2005) *Building a Memory: Preventing Harm, Reducing Risks and Improving Patient Safety* London: The Stationery Office.

NPSA (2006) *Exploring Incidents, Improving Safety: A Guide to Root Cause Analysis* available at www.msnpsa.nhs.uk.

O'Brien-Pallas, L., Duffield, L. and Hayes, L. (2006) Do we really understand how to retain nurses? *Journal of Nursing Management* 14: 262–270.

Oermann, M.H. and Huber, D. (1999) Patient outcomes: a measure of nursing's value. *American Journal of Nursing* 99(9): 40–48.

OPP (2004) *Changing Times*. Available at www.opp.co.uk.

Parish, C. (2005) Recruitment needs to double to keep pace with retirement rates. *Nursing Standard* 19(33): 8.

Pembrey, S. (1980) *The Ward Sister: The Key to Nursing*. London: RCN.

Phipps, K. (2000) Viewpoint. *British Journal of Clinical Governance* 5.

Polit, D.F. (2004) *Nursing Research: Principles and Methods*, 7th edn, Philadelphia: Lippincott, Williams & Wilkins.

Pothier, D., Monteiro, P., Mooktiar, M. and Shaw, A. (2005) Pilot study to show the loss of important data in nursing handover. *British Journal of Nursing* 14(20):1090–1093.

Picker Institute Europe (2005) *Is the NHS Getting Better or Worse? An In-depth Look at the Views of Nearly a Million Patients between 1998 and 2004* Oxford: Picker Institute Europe.

Rafferty, A.M., Clarke, S.P., Coles, J., Ball, J., James, P., McKee, M. and Aiken, L. H. (2006) Outcomes of variation in hospital nurse staffing in English hospitals: Cross-sectional analysis of survey data and discharge records. *International Journal of Nursing Studies* 44(2): 175–82.

RCN (1997) *Health and Safety at Work 6: Shifting the Balance: Towards the Best Practice in Shift Working and Patient Care* London: RCN.

RCN (2002) *Working Well* London: RCN.

RCN (2003) *Defining Nursing* London: RCN.

RCN (2004) *The Future Nurse: The Future Patient* London: RCN.

RCN (2005a) *Working with Care: Improving Working Relationships in Healthcare: Self Assessment Tools for Healthcare Teams* London: RCN.

RCN (2005b) *Past Trends, Future Imperfect? A Review of the Nursing Labour Market in 2004–5* London: RCN.

RCN (2005c) *A Multiple Case Study Evaluation of the RCN Clinical Leadership Programme in England* London: RCN.

RCN (2006) *Setting Safe Nurse Staffing Levels* London: RCN.

Reed, J. and McCormak, B. (2005) The involvement of service users in care, services and policy: comments and implications for nursing development. *International Journal of Older People Nursing* 14(3a): 41–42.

Reid, B., Townson, R., Renton, H. and Shiel, A. (2002) A trial of patient-centred drug administration. *Nursing Times* 98(37): 36–38.

Rogers, A.E., Hwang, W., Scott, L.D., Aiken, L.H. and Dinges, D.F. (2004) The working hours of hospital staff nurses and patient safety *Health Affairs* 23:202–212.

Rowe, A.J. and Mason, R.O. (1987) *Managing with Style: A Guide to Understanding, Assessing and Improving Decision-Making* San Francisco: Jossey-Bass.

Runcimann, W.B. and Merry, A. (2003) A tragic death: a time to blame or a time to learn? *Quality and Safety in Healthcare* 12: 321–322.

Scally, G. and Donaldson, L.J. (1998) Clinical governance and the drive for quality improvement in the new NHS in England. *British Medical Journal* 317: 61–65.

SCOPME (1998) *An Enquiry into Mentoring: Supporting Doctors and Dentists at Work* London: SCOPME.

Scottish Executive (2000) *Our National Health: A Plan for Action, A Plan for Change* Edinburgh: Scottish Executive.

Sexton, A., Chan, C., Elliott, M., Stuart, J., Jayasuriya, R. and Crookes, P. (2004) Nursing handovers: do we really need them? *Journal of Nursing Management* 12(1): 37–42.

Smith, L., McAllister, L. and Crawford, C. (2002) Mentoring benefits and issues for public health nurses. *Public Health Nursing* 18(2): 101–107.

Steven, A. (1999) Named nursing: in whose best interest? *Journal of Advanced Nursing* 29(2): 341–347.

Strachota, E., Normandin, P., O'Brien, N., Clary, M. and Krukow, B. (2003) Reasons registered nurses leave or change employment status. *Journal of Nursing Administration* 33(2): 111–117.

Strebler, M. (2004) *Why Tackle Poor Performance?* Brighton: Institute For Employment Studies.

Thurgood, G. (1995) Verbal handover reports: what skills are needed? *British Journal of Nursing* 4(12): 720–722.

Tierney, A.J. (1998) Nursing models: extant or extinct? *Journal of Advanced Nursing* 28(1): 77–85.

Improving patient outcomes

Torjuul, K., and Sorlie, V. (2006) Nursing is different than medicine: ethical difficulties in the process of care in surgical units. *Journal of Advanced Nursing* 56(4): 404–413.

Tuckman, B.W. (1965) Developmental sequence in small groups. *Psychological Bulletin* 63: 384–399.

Tutton, E.M.M. (2005) Patient participation on a ward for frail older people. *Journal of Advanced Nursing* 50(2): 143–152.

Watkins, S. (1993) Bedside manner. *Nursing Times* 89(29): 42–43.

Wells, A. (2005) Philosophy or fairy tale? *Practice Development in Healthcare* 4(1): 49.

Werner, J.M. and DeSimone, R.L. (2005) *Human Resource Development* Cincinnati, Ohio: South-Western College Publishing.

West, E., Rafferty, A. M. and Lankshear, A. (2004) *The Future Nurse: Evidence of the Impact of Registered Nurses* London: RCN.

Wilson, J.L. (2002) The impact of shift patterns on healthcare professionals. *Journal of Nursing Management* 10(4): 211–219.

Wimpenny, P. (2002) The meaning of models of nursing to practising nurses. *Journal of Advanced Nursing* 40(3): 346–354.

Yoder, L.H. (1995) Staff nurses' career development relationships and self-reports of professionalism, job satisfaction, and intent to stay. *Nursing Research* 44(5): 290–297.

Index

Index